Thorsons Guide to Health

Arthritis

Other titles in this series:

Thorsons Natural Health

Arthritis

LEON CHAITOW

Thorsons

An Imprint of HarperCollins*Publishers*

Thorsons

An Imprint of HarperCollins*Publishers*

77–85 Fulham Palace Road,

Hammersmith, London W6 8JB

First published by Thorsons 1987

This revised, enlarged and reset edition 1997

10 9 8 7 6 5 4 3 2 1

© Leon Chaitow 1997

Leon Chaitow asserts the moral right to
be identified as the author of this work.
A catalogue record for this book
is available from the British Library

ISBN 0 7225 3562 7

Printed and bound in Great Britain by
Caledonian International Book Manufacturing Ltd, Glasgow

Contents

Note to Reader

Before following the self-help advice given in this book, readers are urged to give careful consideration to the nature of their particular health problem, and to consult a competent physician if in any doubt. This book should not be regarded as a substitute for professional medical treatment, and whilst every care is taken to ensure the accuracy of the content, the author and the publishers cannot accept legal responsibility for any problem arising out of the experimentation with the methods described.

Introduction

Most people, by the time they are middle aged (say 40 upwards) will have some degree of osteoarthritis in their body. The most likely sites are in the weight-bearing joints of the body: hips, knees, spine, etc. In many cases the only sign of the condition will be a degree of stiffness, and seldom much pain. Pain, however, will become evident if these compromised joints are asked to perform tasks which are no longer easy for them.

Man has been described as a two-legged creature with a backache. The backache suffered by most middle-aged people relates to some degree of osteoarthritis, and the reasons for the human animal's back problems are thought to relate to a failure to adapt fully to the upright position.

In evolutionary terms, the way the spine was carried when, in distant history, man's forebears were on all fours provided the spinal structures with adequate support and shock-absorbing capacity.

A leading spinal researcher, Professor Korr of Texas University School of Osteopathic Medicine, has noted the change thus: 'The spine of man is a perfect cantilever bridge (when in the all-fours position) and has been turned through a 90-degree angle and is now an unstable skyscraper'. We are apparently faced with nature's uncompleted adaptation as a cause of our weak backs. This is a major reason for the development of osteoarthritis, as the stresses and strains of use in modern life impose their wear and tear on the joints of this region.

Failure to adapt to other aspects of life, nutritional in the main, may well lie behind some cases of rheumatoid arthritis, which has elements in its make-up of allergy and self-allergy (autoimmune disease). In many cases this has been shown to be the result of a combination of nutrient deficiency and intolerance to certain foods, notably those which have been introduced to man's diet in comparatively recent history, such as grains and dairy produce.

Some of the strategies available to us in dealing with these problems in a self-help manner are explained in later chapters. They are not always easy answers, though, and in some cases the best that can be hoped for is a coping strategy rather than cure, since once joint surfaces are damaged beyond a certain point they cannot be expected to regenerate. Safe pain-relief, improvement of mobility and reduction of inflammatory processes are the major elements in self-help methods. These entail both externally and internally applied measures involving nutrients and herbal substances.

Medical care is largely palliative in these conditions. Most of the drugs used in rheumatology are dangerous, some extremely so, including cortisone and the common anti-inflammatory drugs (over-the-counter and prescription medication to kill pain and reduce inflammation), some of which have been discredited because of the widespread side-effects they have caused. Surgery offers a chance of a new lease of life in many cases of joint destruction, and the technical brilliance of these operations should be applauded, even if they are patching up damage rather than curing it. Such methods are most successful in hips and knees, and to a large extent finger joints damaged beyond repair by arthritic processes. Surgery offers little for people with multiple joint problems, however.

Prevention must remain the major objective, and this is best achieved by a balanced diet, good body use and the ability to cope well with stress factors. Attention to the overall use of the body in work, home and play, in terms of minimizing stresses and strains on the mechanical component generally and the spine in particular, is most important in this respect. Advice and attention from a qualified osteopathic or chiropractic practitioner, on the basis of check-ups every six months even if there are no problems, is a wise precaution to take, and should be adopted for children from their early years. In this manner much mechanical damage can be avoided and much suffering prevented.

In the following chapters we will be examining the major areas of arthritic change, osteoarthritis and rheumatoid arthritis. There are many other conditions which can loosely be grouped together as arthritic or rheumatic, but these two major areas are the ones we will concentrate upon. The self-help measures outlined can well be adapted to most joint problems, however, since they are not harmful if performed in the manner advised.

Self-help involves effort and continuity. Few of the measures mentioned will do much if performed only once or twice, or if not continued over a long period. This is especially true of nutritional methods, which are literally trying to alter the biochemistry of the body. This is seldom achieved speedily, and should be viewed as an on-going pattern if relief is to be found for chronic problems.

All healing comes from within; the measures in this book attempt to deal with all aspects, physical and mental, to offer the processes and ingredients which can assist the healing processes to the greatest extent possible, and to provide relief where healing is not fully possible.

1
What Is Arthritis?

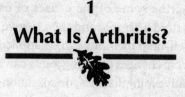

Before arthritic sufferers can help themselves to recover from or control arthritis, it is useful for them to understand the term. All animals with a back bone, including man, are prone to arthritis and apparently have been throughout history. Evidence of this condition can be found in prehistoric man and also in the skeletons of the dinosaurs.

Osteoarthritis is a condition rather than a disease and it can have a variety of causes. Rheumatoid arthritis, however, is a disease; it and osteoarthritis are not in any way related except that in the late stages of rheumatoid arthritis, when the active inflammation of the joints is 'burned-out', some osteoarthritic changes develop. The need to clarify just which type of arthritis is present will become apparent when we understand just how different the two types are. There are of course a large number of conditions which carry the label 'arthritis', but in the main these are rare, so it is our task to describe some of the causes of osteoarthritis and rheumatoid arthritis, and then to give suggestions as to how self-help methods can be applied.

All arthritic changes affecting joints can be described as degenerative joint diseases, or conditions. The causes lie in a variety of factors including heredity, ageing, wear and tear, posture, occupation, nutrition, allergies, injury, infection, body weight, inflammatory factors, and hormonal alterations – or any combination of these and other factors. Bearing in mind that we are discussing different and distinct conditions, and that the word 'arthritis' can be applied to quite separate entities, we will begin by examining osteoarthritis, the all-pervasive form.

Osteoarthritis

Osteoarthritis is that form of arthritis which is most responsible for incapacity, loss of time from work, and general disability. It affects mainly the hips, knees, spine and fingers (fingers and knees are more affected in women, hips and the spine in men).

Osteoarthritis can manifest itself as early as the late teens, and is probably present (although usually with few or no symptoms) in nearly everyone by the time they are in their seventies. It is a local condition which means that its development is not usually accompanied by systemic changes in the blood or in the body as a whole. It appears in one or several joints co-incidentally since, quite obviously, if the state of the individual's body is such as to allow the development of degenerative changes in one joint, it will be the same for any other joints that may be similarly under postural, mechanical or traumatic stress.

What actually takes place in a joint which is becoming osteoarthritic is a wearing away of the smooth, polished cartilage, which is the gliding interface lying between the bones of a joint. This wearing process tends to expose the underlying bone to wear and pressure. Particles of damaged cartilage and bone become irritated and ultimately inflamed as a result, and there is a protective effort on the part of the body to repair, splint or cushion the damaged area. This involves enzymes, blood cells, etc., and regardless of the initial cause or the actual bodily response, the underlying cartilage, and the fluid in which it is bathed, begin to show signs of change.

The body then makes a defensive attempt to reinforce the damaged cartilage structure, and fluid from the joint may be unable to sustain its nutritive role to help maintain and regenerate the cartilage. This failure to maintain and repair the cartilage may take place during a major inflammatory stage, or at times of repetitive overuse associated with minor inflammation of the area.

As the cartilage develops increasing signs of wear, and the underlying bone becomes irritated, there is a proliferation of the bone as new cells are laid down to deal with the injury. The new bone forms outcroppings known as osteophytes; these grow larger as the cartilage becomes increasingly worn away.

By this stage the structure and shape of the end of the bone will have begun to alter and there will be alterations too in the degree and range of free movement in the joint.

This more restricted movement may result in greater stress as the individual attempts to use a severely affected joint. There are therefore waves of inflammation, each of which further aggravates the wear and tear process, with consequent desperate local attempts by the body to splint and rebuild the damaged joint surface.

This results in the vicious cycle of damage and pain repeating itself over again. Once movement has been severely compromised the repetition of this cycle declines, because effectively the body will have prevented movement and use. By this stage lumpy, deformed joints are often evident. These are frequently unstable, but may be relatively painless, unless attempts to use them are made. This represents a typical development of an osteoarthritic joint which may take months or even years to reach a stable, but almost totally damaged state.

A joint may, however, never deteriorate to such an extent; instead changes may be minor and the limitations in the movement of the joint remain virtually unnoticed. For example, X-rays of most adults over 40 will show some osteoarthritic changes in their necks. However, most of these individuals will be completely symptom-free. It may therefore be assumed that the process of repair and new bone growth, which the body institutes in response to wear of the joint surface, is nearly always successfully achieved.

From this sequence we can see that this form of arthritis is often actually helpful, in that it protects the damaged joint surface from greater destruction. It is only when this process is accompanied by excessive inflammation and repeated laying down of new bone growth that extreme limitation occurs. Thus the factors which need to be examined are those that determine the degree of inflammation and the ability of the body to respond adequately without going beyond what is desirable in the way of repair and splinting.

Self-healing

If most people have pain-free joints which show signs of osteoarthritis, it must be assumed that this is part of the marvellous self-maintenance mechanism of the body. After all, the body would cease to function adequately if it did not attempt to repair the initial stages of cartilage wear, for then the cartilage would simply wear away and the bone underlying it would do the same.

The response of the body has to be sufficient to protect the underlying bone so that further damage is avoided and joint movement is not impeded. If osteoarthritis is tackled at an early stage and the body is assisted in the task of repair, then there is every chance that the amount of damage can be contained, and a virtually symptomless stage reached. For this to happen the underlying causes need to be found and then rectified. This may entail losing weight, improving posture or reducing habitual or occupational stress. It also entails providing the body generally, and the joint specifically, with the optimum environment for repair.

This means that the nutritional status of the individual must be at its optimum so that the nutrients vital for repair are present. It also means that local circulation and muscle tone must be at their best, as both are necessary for the repair and maintenance of joints. This calls for a variety of exercises to improve muscle tone and enhance circulatory efficiency.

By removing the underlying causes, helping the repair process, enhancing the efficiency of circulation and improving muscle tone, most osteoarthritic conditions will be improved, and often become symptom-free. (This is provided that the damage of joints has not advanced beyond a point of no return.)

Even if damage has progressed beyond such a stage, however, there is still much that can be done firstly to prevent the progression of the condition, and then hopefully to reduce pain, stiffness and associated disability as much as possible.

NOTE: The self-help measures outlined below are not meant to be undertaken in isolation from responsible professional advice and care, but are suggested as useful tactics to enhance whatever else is being done to and for you.

Understanding Homeostasis

It is absolutely vital for anyone afflicted with a chronic illness to hold on to the fact that their body is a self-healing mechanism, that since broken bones mend and cuts usually heal, and since most health disturbances – from infections to digestive disturbances – get better with or without treatment (often faster without!) – that in a healthy state there must be a constant process for normalization and health promotion in operation. This is called homeostasis.

The homeostatic functions (which include the immune system) can become overwhelmed by too many tasks and demands, because of (perhaps) any or all of the following:

- nutritional deficiencies
- accumulated toxic material (environmental

pollution, either as food or inhaled, in medication, previous or current use of drugs, etc.)
- emotional stress
- recurrent or current infections
- allergies
- modified functional ability due to age or inborn factors or acquired habits involving poor posture, breathing imbalances and/or sleep disturbances, and so on …

At a certain point in time the adaptive homeostatic mechanisms break down and frank illness – disease – appears. At this time the body needs help – treatment – and this can take the form of either:

a. Reducing the load which is impacting the body by taking away as many of the undesirable factors as possible – by avoiding allergens, improving posture and breathing, learning stress coping tactics, improving diet, using supplements if called for, helping to normalize sleep and circulatory function, introducing a detoxification programme, dealing with infections – and generally trying to keep the pressure off the defence mechanisms while they focus on the current urgent repair needs.
b. Enhancing, improving and modulating the defence and repair processes by a variety of means, mainly non-specific.

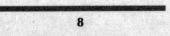

c. Treating the symptoms – while making sure that we are doing nothing to add further to the burden on the defence mechanisms.

Not all of the possible beneficial methods which are available need to be used, because once the load on the repair processes is reduced sufficiently a degree of normal homeostatic function is automatically restored and self-healing processes become more active.

This means that in any given case it is necessary to focus attention on what seems the likeliest and easiest targets (perhaps using a team approach in which more than one therapy is being used) which will achieve this desirable end.

In one person this may call for dietary modification and stress reduction, while in another enhancement of immune function via avoidance of allergens, use of hydrotherapy and reduction in symptoms using simple bodywork and exercise.

The self-help methods that we will be discussing in subsequent chapters are ones which can easily be applied at home. Of course there are specialized treatments which do not fall within the scope of self-help. These include the use of osteopathic and chiropractic manipulation to help normalize body mechanics; acupuncture to relieve pain and stiffness and enhance circulation; physiotherapy (including ultrasonic therapy) to help contain localized inflammation; surgical measures to replace damaged joints; and splinting and support for damaged joints, such as the knee, which may have become unstable.

Such measures, although lying beyond the scope of this book, should be borne in mind. But a note of caution should be added: the standard medical therapy for osteoarthritis, involving the use of anti-inflammatory drugs, has been shown to cause much suffering and, in rare cases, even death. Many anti-arthritic drugs which have arrived in a blaze of publicity have been withdrawn after a few years under a cloud of suspicion that they involve far more suffering than ever they relieved. Aspirin is still the safest of all anti-arthritic drugs, for all its shortcomings.

Drugless Healing

The methods we will be discussing do not involve drugs. Should the individual with arthritis be taking drugs, under medical supervision, there is no reason whatever why the methods outlined here should not be employed, for they are supportive of the body and have no bad side-effects.

Having found a programme which helps to minimize the causes of the condition, and which enhances the defensive ability of the body, it may well be that drugs can eventually (with your doctor's agreement) be phased out.

Self-help is the aim. This does of course call for some effort on the patient's part. Intelligent cooperation in any programme is essential. It is not advisable to undertake diets and exercises grudgingly or half-heartedly. Rather, see the good sense of what is involved and resolutely undertake whatever needs to be done, with the long-term view of better health, greater mobility and the use of presently compromised joints. This is the way to begin helping the body to recover.

Rheumatoid Arthritis Overview

Before looking at any of the individual methods that will help the body, we must consider the other major arthritic condition, namely rheumatoid arthritis. This is a chronic, usually progressive inflammatory disorder of the joints. It is more common in women than men and occurs at any age, but usually between the ages of 25 and 55. The condition usually involves bilateral (both sides of the body) symptoms, although very occasionally it may appear on one side only; if so, it usually involves the knees.

The symmetrical, two-sided, development of symptoms is distinctive of rheumatoid arthritis, since osteoarthritis commonly affects only one joint.

The inflammatory process in rheumatoid arthritis is usually progressive and, depending upon the severity of the attack, can completely destroy the joints' ability to function, leaving them swollen and distorted. The affected joints will also be warm or even hot, reddened and tender, at least during the active phase of the disease. There is a characteristic stiffness in the mornings which tends to last half an hour or so, but which may last for hours. At the outset it is the pain which limits movement, but as time passes the supporting tissues of the joints change and fibrosis occurs, which limits the elasticity of the area.

Limitation of movement may become profound and ankylosis may occur. This means that bones which normally have a degree of movement between them actually become fused. Initially, the joints most commonly affected are those of the hands, feet, wrists and knees. Later this may spread to the elbows, shoulders, ankles, hips and collar bone. Sometimes the jaw may become affected. Unlike osteoarthritis, in rheumatoid arthritis the spine is rarely affected, and if it is, usually only the neck region is involved.

If the fingers are affected by rheumatoid arthritis, in the early stages the joints swell and become spindle-shaped. This often clears after a few years as the condition progresses to other areas. There is often a deformity of the fingers so that there is a twisting outwards of the joints to produce a deviation from the normal position. This is combined with damage to the tendons which guide the joints. This may result in distortion producing abnormal flexion of the fingers so that it becomes impossible to bring the fingertips together. This makes the lifting of small objects very difficult and sometimes impossible. Such distortion is possible in any affected joint, and the disability and progressive pain which this produces makes it a nightmare of endurance.

The onset of rheumatoid arthritis is frequently accompanied by loss of weight and appetite, fatigue and unaccountable fever and sweats. There may be obvious nodules, which can be felt under the skin, and there is often generalized aching and stiffness, not at first localized to the joints themselves. At first the sufferer may be aware only of the involvement of the joints. However, many other systemic changes may occur, including inflammation of the blood vessels, weakness and wasting of muscles, and inflammation of the heart muscle (in about 40 per cent of cases). Breathing and sometimes the eyes may be affected; the lymph glands and spleen may become swollen. Anaemia usually accompanies this disease, despite the fact that the body is not short of iron. It seems that there is an accompanying inability to utilize the iron supply adequately. Rheumatoid arthritis is a systemic disease in that the whole body is involved, and this makes it different from osteoarthritis in which only specific joints are affected.

Causes

The causes of rheumatoid arthritis are unknown, although the processes that occur are minutely understood. The major theory suggests that rheumatoid arthritis is due to an unnatural behaviour of the body's immune system so that, for reasons which are unclear, the defence mechanisms actually attack the body tissues, in this case articular joint tissues. Thus, the very elements which are designed to protect the body attack it. Why this should happen is uncertain, but it seems probable that a number of factors must be present simultaneously to account for it. Some of the 'unorthodox' theories regarding the cause of this disease will be discussed later.

Statistics confirm that, of any 100 rheumatoid arthritis sufferers:

- 15 will have only a short-lived disease which will remit of its own accord, with no treatment, and leave very little permanent damage.
- A further 25 will have episodes which persist for some time (perhaps months or even years), but will also remit, leaving few after-effects apart from slight joint distortion and a little stiffness.
- A further 50 will have persistent symptoms. They will suffer periods of distress interspersed with periods of remission, gradually leading to deformity and varying degrees of disability.

- The remaining 10 will suffer the relentless progression of the disease, usually quite unresponsive to any treatment, and leading to complications and probable wheelchair confinement.

If remission is going to occur spontaneously, then this usually takes place in the first year, especially if the disease had an acute onset. In general, men have a better chance of remission than women, especially if the disease begins before the age of 45. If there are manifestations of rheumatoid arthritis in areas other than the joints, the prognosis is less good. This is also true if there is X-ray evidence of erosion of the bone surface in affected joints.

The signs that identify rheumatoid arthritis include the following:

- stiffness in the mornings, with pain on movement in at least one joint
- swelling of at least one joint; more probably of the same joint on both sides of the body
- nodules which can be felt over prominent bones or near joints
- apart from these signs there are distinctive bone changes, visible on X-ray, showing inflammation as well as detectable changes in the blood.

The greater the number of symptoms which are manifest, the greater the chances that the condition is rheumatoid arthritis. (The above symptoms must be present for at least six weeks continuously for a positive diagnosis to be made. Shorter periods are probably not the result of rheumatoid arthritis.)

The self-help programme designed to alleviate the symptoms and improve the general health of the sufferer will be described later. Some of the advice which will be offered is applicable to both rheumatoid arthritis and osteoarthritis: for instance, in both cases an inflamed joint can be helped by hydrotherapy. On the other hand, not all treatments are suitable for both conditions and specific advice for rheumatoid arthritic conditions will also be given.

In order to cope with a problem which manifestly involves all aspects of the body it is necessary to advise a reform of the whole pattern of life. This usually includes adequate rest and exercise, nutritional reform, specific supplementation, psychological reorientation and guided imagery, special hydrotherapy measures and the use of helpful herbal and other non-toxic substances.

Allergy as a Factor

One area of health care which needs careful evaluation is that of allergy or food intolerance. It has been demonstrated that some arthritis (osteo- and rheumatoid) patients are in fact displaying a marked reaction against particular foods, and that when these are removed from the diet a dramatic improvement is possible. This is not by any means always the case, but it is desirable to reassess the food that one eats as it relates to the chemical additives which enter the body. Thus a key aspect of a self-help programme is the detoxification of the body which effectively rids the system of any toxic encumbrances which may contribute to arthritis. For instance, this involves the use of methods which ensure a regular bowel function. Other methods will be discussed in subsequent chapters. Some experts have suggested that the combination of allergic reactions to foods and chemical and toxic factors may be the ultimate cause of the faulty immune reaction which leads the body to 'attack' itself.

A large number of other so-called rheumatoid or arthritic conditions exist which are not dealt with in this book. These include gout and all the soft tissue conditions so often lumped together as 'fibrositis and rheumatism'. Measures for self-help and professional care of the latter are covered in full in my book *Fibromyalgia and Muscle Pain* (Thorsons). There is an overlap between all these conditions and some of the advice in this book is applicable to several of them. For instance, in all cases the detoxification of the body and the removal of stress are important factors and greatly contribute to the body's self-healing ability.

2
The Causes of Osteoarthritis

The way we use our body, day in and day out, greatly affects its wear and tear. Posture and habitual use determine the degree of repetitive strain imposed upon joints. Habits of use generally begin in infancy, and so are not particularly easy to correct in adult life. The human spine has been aptly described as a superb cantilever bridge which has been inadequately adapted for use as a skyscraper. The main factor which constantly produces strain on the body, and the spine in particular, is gravity. If the spine is not correctly balanced, strains are imposed upon certain of the articulating surfaces.

If we consider the other everyday strains which are added to the stresses caused by poor posture, then we can appreciate the great number of strains to which our bodies are subject. Footwear is a major cause of strain. High heels, especially, throw the weight of the body forward of its centre of gravity. This results in alterations in muscular patterns which in turn place increased weight on joints which were never designed for such stresses. The hips, knees, feet and joints of the lower back and pelvis are particularly involved in such strains.

The regular use of poorly designed furniture is another factor in unnatural wear and tear. Chairs which provide inadequate support, or which are too low or too high in relation to body size and particular activities (e.g. computer use) contribute to body strain. Newer designs of chairs allow for a degree of kneeling, and consequently provide a far more desirable spinal contour than traditional chairs. Such chairs are now increasingly becoming available from specialist 'back shops' and the better of the office supply companies.

Beds that are too soft, work surfaces that are the wrong height, or working conditions which impose undesirable stresses contribute further to repetitive muscular and joint strains. In addition, weight-bearing joints are exposed to undue stress if the body weight is above normal, and also if weight carrying or lifting is a regular feature of daily life.

Given that the above factors contribute significantly to osteoarthritic problems, they need to be carefully considered. Is there a degree of overweight? Are there repetitive daily habits which might be unduly straining joints and muscles? Are there habits of posture related to occupation (e.g. typing, hairdressing, lifting) which cause stress? Are there repetitive activities (e.g. sport or hobbies) which might be adding to the strain of joints? Is posture satisfactory? What changes can be made to reduce the stresses that might result from any of the above?

Less obvious factors might be considered. Sitting with legs crossed is a common cause of undue lower back and hip joint torsion and strain; standing habitually with the body weight on one leg is another. Both may result from a pelvic or spinal imbalance which in turn has resulted in one leg appearing to be longer than the other. This should be assessed and dealt with by a qualified osteopathic or chiropractic practitioner. Habits which favour one side of the body should be eliminated. One such habit is the tucking of a telephone between the ear and the shoulder. If this is a common habit, it may result in strain on the neck region with consequent aggravation of arthritic changes which are all too common in that area.

Observation of our daily habits can help us to evaluate those which are unduly stressful, and we can begin to eliminate them. For instance, loss of surplus weight is beneficial, and dealing with apparent or real imbalances, such as short-leg problems, is also useful. Frequently, however, osteoarthritic changes may well be established by the time we become aware of such factors, and changes in lifestyle may not eliminate the problems. Yet these changes can be important in reducing pain and discomfort, and in slowing or checking progression of the condition. It may be useful to look at ourselves in photographs, so as to check for habitual tilting of the head or other obvious postural imbalances. Look to see whether eyes, ears and shoulders are level. Such factors provide clues to deviations in the contour of the spine, and these deviations may benefit from regular stretching exercises, as well as from attention by a practitioner skilled in spine and body mechanics.

Long before joint problems become manifest there will have been a tendency for the soft tissues of the region to become stiffer and tighter than usual. Often this is taken simply as part of the ageing process and so is endured. Yet, were attention paid to early stiffness in muscles and soft tissues, there is a good chance that the insidious onset of joint dysfunction and ultimate osteoarthritic change might have been prevented. It is important that after any injury (such as a fall, jar or blow) that leaves a region less than fully free and mobile, attention should be given by a suitably qualified practitioner. Sporting injuries often become arthritic many years later, simply as a result of inadequate attention at the time of injury. Motor car accidents, especially those involving violent jarring (such as whiplash of the neck) can have similar long-term effects. If the soft tissues are given attention soon after such injuries, then joint damage is more likely to be avoided.

Emotional strain, which produces a tensing and contracting of groups of muscles, is another cause of osteoarthritic changes. It can impair joint movement and circulation. Such effects of emotional stress may be overcome by regular stretching exercises, such as those used in yoga, as well as stress-reduction methods. These methods are discussed in the next chapter.

3
Self-help for Arthritis

Stretching Exercises

The following stretching exercises are recommended as part of a general prevention programme. They may not be entirely suitable for all arthritic sufferers. If they hurt then they are being done too enthusiastically and require modification. If they do not hurt during performance, and leave the area more supple, then they are desirable. Specific exercises can be used for specific areas, however the following are meant for general stretching and limbering. They are appropriate for individuals with osteoarthritis, rheumatoid arthritis or stiffness, as long as no pain results.

These exercises are meant to produce general effects. To start with, do the following movements three times each. After a few days increase to 10 times each.

1. Stand up straight with your feet apart and your hands clasped behind your back. Allow yourself to bend forward from the hips as far as is comfortable. Use no effort but try to allow the weight of the upper body to stretch you forwards. Feel the stretch up the back of your legs and especially behind the knees. This exercise is not repeated. You simply hold the position for half a minute; breathe slowly and deeply and allow the stretch to reach its maximum. As the days go by allow the time in this position to increase to 3 minutes. This stretches the hamstrings, helps the muscular supporting structures of the pelvis and improves abdominal tone, but it is important to breathe slowly and deeply all the while.

2. For the following exercise you may, at first, need to hold on to a solid object such as a heavy table, in order not to lose your balance. If you can do it unaided, so much the better.

   With feet about 12–15 inches (30–38 cm) apart and standing up straight, slowly go into a squatting position, trying to keep your heels on the floor. If this is not possible then go just as far as you can into the squat without raising your heels. As you squat, stretch your arms forward and lean forward from the waist to maintain balance. If you feel you are toppling backwards you may need to balance yourself by holding on to a table or some other heavy object. When you are at the fullest limit of your squat give a few gentle up and down 'jigs' as though you are trying to tuck your tail between your legs. Rise and repeat.

This exercise tones the hamstrings, acts as a general stimulant to circulation and muscle tone in the pelvic area, and stretches the lower back. When it becomes easy to perform you can vary it by using the more advanced technique of interlocking the fingers behind the neck as you start (head facing straight ahead). At the end of each deep squat rise to your feet slowly, and as you do so stretch the hands (still interlocked) towards the ceiling, pressing open palms as far up-wards as possible. This is further enhanced by breathing in deeply as you stretch upwards. Repeat 3 to 10 times.

3. The following variations on chair exercises are designed to achieve general stretching of the upper part of the body, without strain. First, sit on an ordinary dining chair, feet together and hands clasped behind the back. Bend forward from the waist with the hands stretching backwards and upwards as far as possible. Your trunk should be leaning as far forward as possible, so that your nose is as close to your knees as it can get. The hands should stretch up and back and be held there for 5 to 10 seconds, as you breathe in and out. Sit up and repeat.

4. After doing this a number of times separate your feet so that there is a wide gap between your knees. Repeat the exercise, but instead of bending straight

forwards, bend towards each knee alternately. This time keep the hands clasped behind the back without stretching them backwards. Repeat several times in each direction, holding for a full cycle of breathing.

5. Sit straight up in the chair, feet together and arms extended sideways, palms downwards. Breathe in and turn the palms upwards and at the same time stretch the arms backwards so that you feel the shoulder blades coming towards each other. Relax and breathe out as you let the arms resume their original position. Repeat.

6. Sitting, place your hands behind your neck, or rest the fingertips on the shoulders, whichever is the more comfortable. Slowly rotate the shoulders so that your arms are moving in a gentle circle (as though you are drawing circles with your elbows). Repeat in each direction several times. You should try to achieve maximum stretch as the elbows circle, so that they go back, then down, then forward, then up as far as possible in each direction of circling.

Relaxation

This method of relaxation should be introduced at the outset of any self-help approach to healing. Whilst learning the technique, arrange to have two free periods per day, each of 5 to 15 minutes' duration. Find a quiet room where you know you will not be disturbed.

Rest on your back, with head and shoulders slightly raised, and pillows under the knees to take the strain off them and your back. Rest your hands on the upper abdomen, close your eyes and settle down in a comfortable position. Ensure that there is nothing to distract your attention, such as sunlight, a clock, or pets. Sitting in a reclining position is also suitable, and many people prefer this to lying down. Try both and choose whichever is most comfortable.

Deep breathing is of great value in relaxation, particularly during the initial stages. It is partly carried out through the autonomic nervous system and partly through the central nervous system. The autonomic nervous system is that which controls vital functions, endocrine (hormone) secretions and emotions. By controlling one's breathing, one can influence all these functions and, for a short time, take over conscious responsibility from them. Breathing is the only automatic function which one is easily able to control.

The aim is to breathe slowly, deeply and rhythmically. You cannot expect to do this perfectly from the start – it might take weeks. Inhale through the nose slowly and deeply. The abdomen, on which the hands are resting, should rise gently as the breathing begins. An awareness of this rising and falling of the abdomen is important to establish that the diaphragm is being used properly. Inhalation should be slow, unforced and unhurried. Whilst breathing in, slowly and silently, count to 4, 5 or 6. When the inhalation is complete, pause for 2 or 3 seconds, then slowly exhale through the nose. As you exhale, you should feel the abdomen slowly falling. While breathing out count again to 4, 5 or 6. The exhalation should take at least as long as the inhalation.

There should be no sense of strain when breathing. If at first you feel that you have breathed to your fullest capacity by a count of 3, work gradually to improve on this. Try to slow down the rhythm until a slow count of 5 or 6 is possible, both on inhalation and exhalation, with a pause of 2 or 3 second between. Remember to start each breath with an upwards push of the abdomen. With the mind thus occupied on the mechanics of breathing and the rhythmic counting, there is little scope for thinking about anything else. Nevertheless, initially at least, extraneous thoughts will intrude. This pattern of breathing should be repeated 15 to 20 times and, since each cycle should take about 15 seconds, this exercise should occupy a total of about 5 minutes.

Once slow, rhythmic breathing becomes well established it is useful to introduce a pattern of thoughts during different phases of the breathing cycle. For example, on inhalation try to sense a feeling of warmth and energy entering the body with the air. On exhaling, sense a feeling of sinking and settling deeper into the supporting surface. An overall sense of warmth and heaviness accompanying the repetitive breathing cycle will enhance relaxation. Physiologically, this exercise will slow down the heart rate, reduce sympathetic nervous activity, relax tense muscles and allow a chance for the balancing, restorative, parasympathetic nervous functions to operate. It calms the mind as well.

After a few weeks begin to introduce specific images into your thought patterns of any painful or restricted areas being freed and loosened. 'See' the muscles letting go and feel the circulation coursing through the tissues. With this image try to see any affected areas as moving and pain-free. Spend a minute or so on any joint or area that is a problem. Visualization of this sort has a definite physiological effect and deserves repetition daily.

The use of regular stretching exercises, and of a general relaxation method, is an important first step in getting the body harnessed to the task of recovery. If walking is not a problem then regular walking should also be introduced. At least 20 minutes every other day (more if possible) should be the aim. As an alternative, swimming offers the safest and most beneficial exercise for anyone with either osteoarthritis or rheumatoid arthritis.

Exercise during periods of acute arthritic pain should, however, be limited. Slow movements which stretch tight muscles and tone weak ones painlessly are highly desirable in such circumstances. The level of activity desirable should be tailored to your particular condition, so it is not possible to be specific here. However, walking or swimming should be brisk enough in general to leave the individual slightly out of breath, but not sufficient to cause any distress or pain. By regular exercise the same distance can be covered in a progressively shorter time as fitness improves; or better still the distance covered in the time allotted can gradually be increased.

Stretching and relaxation exercises, together with walking or swimming, will improve general circulation, including the flow of lymphatic fluid, which acts as the main channel of detoxification of the body. In this way specific and local changes will take place, despite the general nature of the exercises.

Muscle Energy Techniques

More localized attention can be given to any restricted joint by using modified muscle energy techniques. An osteopathic manoeuvre exists which can be adapted as a self-help method to ease tight and restricted muscles and joints. These exercises are based on the physiological fact that every muscle, or group of muscles, has an opposing or antagonistic muscle, or set of muscles. When one set of muscles is being used, the opposing set is obliged to relax. This means that muscles which have tightened or become stiff and restricted may be eased by making the opposing set of muscles work.

The best way of doing this is through isometric exercises. This means that the muscle that is used is made to work, without any actual movement taking place. If a joint is restricted in movement, for instance if the elbow is difficult to straighten, then it should be gently taken to the comfortable limit, in the direction in which it is restricted. This means that an attempt is made to place the arm in the maximum degree of straightness, without causing pain. At that point the other hand is placed on the forearm (which could be resting on the arm of a chair), so as to restrict the next stage of the operation, which is a firm, steady – not jerky – attempt to bend the arm. The restriction placed on the arm by the other hand should exactly match the effort being made to bend the arm. Thus, of course, no movement should take place. This effort and counter-effort should be maintained for 5 to 10 seconds before a gradual easing of effort is allowed and the arm is rested for a few seconds.

At that point it may be possible, without force or pain, to obtain a little more movement, and the arm may straighten a little more easily. Again the joint should be taken to the limit of the restricted movement and the same procedure adopted as before, with the arm bent, resisted by the counter-pressure of the other hand (but not using your full strength). Allow a period of 5 to 10 seconds during which the pressures exactly match each other before releasing the arm. Then test the joint again to see if a little more of its normal range of movement has been reached.

This method can be used on most joints in the body. However, it cannot always be used on joints which are not easily accessible, for example the spinal joints. The joints of the limbs, shoulder and neck, though, are reasonably accessible and so can be adapted to the above exercise. In some cases there is a better result if, while the joint is being thus treated, there is a slow release of the restricting pressure, so as to allow the joint to move, albeit very slowly, in the direction opposite to the main joint restriction.

The number of times that this can be repeated at any one session depends upon the improvement gained. Once the method has been used with no further movement being gained, it is probably all that is required for that joint at that time. Of course, some joints require that the angle at which the restricted movement is attempted be varied, to help develop movement in several different directions. By varying the angle of resisted effort all the muscles of a joint can be brought into play, little by little. At no time should pain be felt when these procedures are being used. Even if no great increase in the range of movement is achieved, perhaps because of existing joint damage, this exercise will still provide relaxation of the soft tissue structures, which in turn will make the area more comfortable.

These types of exercises are of use in either osteoarthritic or rheumatoid conditions, as well as a wide range of muscular rheumatic and fibrositic states, as long as pain is not precipitated by them. The effort involved should match exactly the comfortable degree of restriction of movement that the free hand or hands can apply.

Trigger Point Self-treatment

In most arthritic patients there exist specific localized areas, in muscles associated with arthritic joints which, when pressed, are sore both locally and also send pain to another area, sometimes quite a distance away. For example, such points are commonly found in the muscles between the shoulder and the neck (trapezius muscles). When pressed, these points hurt locally and often send pain and discomfort to the arm, mid-spine or head. Such points are called trigger points because they trigger pain in a target area. They frequently result in the wrong area being treated. For example, a trapezius trigger can cause a more or less constant pain in the side of the neck and head and if these areas are treated no benefit is likely. Only when the trigger is identified and removed, by one means or another, will the pain in the target area disappear.

There are many ways of dealing with such trigger points, including the use of injections. However, the following treatment is one of the best ways of dealing with a trigger point. Firstly, apply pressure by squeezing or directly pressing on the point for about 10 seconds. Pressure should be just sufficient to relay discomfort to the target area. After 10 seconds ease off for about 5 seconds and then repeat the pressure. Do this 3 or 4 times. Then apply either ice or a cold spray (obtainable from any pharmacy) to the trigger point, with gentle sweeps towards the target area. The chilling should be done in such a way as to cool thoroughly all the tissues between the trigger and the target, without blanching or frosting the skin. This may take anything from 5 to 20 seconds, depending on the size of the area involved.

After the chilling, during which time the ice or the spray is kept constantly moving, the muscles should be gently stretched to their comfortable limit. The muscles should be held there for half a minute or so and then the chilling and stretching should be repeated. This can be done 2 or 3 times, after which the trigger point should be less active. This will become apparent in that less discomfort will be felt.

Triggers can be found in any muscle, and are almost always present when a joint has become restricted. Both the 'muscle energy' method and the chilling and stretching method will help in keeping such muscles and localized areas from becoming unduly troublesome. Regular treatment of this sort can result in a greatly diminished pain level, and an increased mobility of the joints controlled by muscles thus affected. (More information in identifying and dealing with such points can be found in my book *Holistic Pain Relief* [Thorsons].)

Strain/Counterstrain Methods

One of the most successful approaches to treating muscle and joint pain is called strain/counterstrain. In the case of almost any painful condition – acute or chronic – apply the following simple methods and you may be amazed at the relief you get (even if this is only short-lived, as will be the case if the underlying causes have not been eliminated):

1. Gently test the area (muscle, joint) to see which movements cause you discomfort or pain, or which are restricted, carefully noting in which direction movement produces pain or restriction. It is important to note that what you are being asked to observe is *which direction* of movement is restricted or painful – not *where* the pain is felt.

   For example, it might hurt you most to turn your neck to the right and to look upwards, while turning left and looking down might hurt less or not at all.

2. Search, by gentle finger or thumb pressure, for tender or sore points *in the soft tissues (muscles, etc.) which would be working if the opposite movement to that which causes you pain were being performed.*

   In this example these would be the muscles on the left and front of your neck, which are the muscles which would help your head to turn to the left and to bend forwards.

3. Once you have found the most tender point, keep a light pressure on it so that you can use it to guide you in the next stages of the method.

4. Now *very gently and slowly* move the affected area (in this case your head and neck) so that the tenderness goes out of the point on which you are pressing lightly.

   Any movement which causes the pain to increase, either in the neck/head, or on the point you are pressing, is movement in the wrong direction.

   You will find that there is *always* a position of 'maximum ease' in which both (in this example) the neck/head and the tender point will be either pain-free or far less uncomfortable. You have to find that position yourself, but there are general guidelines which can help:

   if the tender point is on the front part of your body you will probably have to bend forward to ease it (as well as using sidebending and rotation in most cases), whereas if the tender point is on the back of your body you may have to bend backwards, as well as making additional 'fine-tuning' movements which may include twisting or sidebending in order to get the tissues into a (relatively) pain-free state.

Remember that the object of your effort is to remove the tenderness from the spot on which you are pressing, but that whatever movements this calls for should not increase pain in the affected area itself (neck/head in this instance), nor create new pain anywhere else. In our example of finding it painful to turn your head right and up, you would search for the tender point in the muscles on the left and front of your neck and upper shoulder area, the very muscles which would need to be active to produce the exact opposite movement. Having found a suitably tender point and holding light pressure on it, you would probably find that by letting your head tilt forward and down with a little turn to the left (and perhaps sidebending to one side or the other while lifting your left shoulder slightly, the pain would vanish from the point. To do this you might need to be lying down, rather than sitting or standing, so that the area is supported.

5. Once you have the position of ease, rest there *for at least a minute* before slowly taking your head/neck back to a neutral position.

The whole area should feel easier and less painful and restricted, and the movement which produced pain before should do so to a far lesser degree – and the tender point should be far less irritable on pressure.

6. You can do the same thing for any painful point you locate.
7. You can use the 'strain/counterstrain' method, exactly as described above, on any tender or sore point in any muscle in the body. If the soreness is chronic the relief may only be short-lived, but if of recent onset the relief can be permanent.

As a further example, the self-treatment of a painful point in the upper trapezius muscle will be described. This is an area which is tender in most people and which causes a lot of problems in people with neck, shoulder and upper back arthritis.

The trapezius muscle runs from the neck to the shoulder; you will find easy access to tender points in it by using a slight 'pinching' grip on the muscle using your thumb and index finger to squeeze the muscle fibres gently until the tender area is found. If pressure is maintained on this tender point for 3 or 4 seconds it might well start to produce a radiating pain in a distant site, probably the head, in which case this tender point is also a trigger point.

Example

To treat the tenderness in the left trapezius you should lie down on the side opposite that which you are treating – in this example, your right side – with your head resting on a cushion. With your right hand, lightly pinch the point, then try altering the position of your left arm, perhaps taking it up and over your head to 'slacken' the muscle you are palpating, or altering your neck position by moving your head backwards a little and slightly sidebending it towards the painful side. 'Fine-tune' the arm and head positions until you reduce the soreness in your pain point (don't pinch it all the time, just intermittently to test whether a new arm and head position is causing it to ease).

Once you find your position of ease, stay in that position for not less than 1 minute.

Slowly return your arm and head to a neutral position, sit up and seek out a tender point in much the same position on the other side. Repeat the exercise.

It is worth re-emphasizing that strain-counterstrain will reduce pain and restriction to some extent in most chronic pain problems, but the results may not last more than an hour or two if fibrotic changes have taken place in the soft tissues. This would call for additional treatment (such as Muscle Energy Technique – described above) from a professional.

How Does this Positional Release Method Work?

a. According to research, in simple terms what seems to be happening when a stressed area of muscle is placed in a position of 'ease' is that nerve-reporting stations, called muscle spindles, 'reset' themselves and so reduce the amount of excessive tension or tone which the muscle is holding. If the muscle was previously in spasm, or even just being held in a state of tension, this would relax and free the tissues, at least for a short while.

b. Additional research has shown that when in a position of 'ease' muscles enjoy a greatly improved blood supply. This means that if the muscle had been relatively short of oxygen before being positioned in this way it would, after the experience, be better oxygenated and nourished, and should therefore be less painful.

Much of the success of the method depends on how long the position of ease is held, which indicates that something is actually happening during that time other than simply being a (relatively) pain-free period – the benefits seem to depend on a combined neural resetting of tone coupled with improved circulation.

Self-massage for Pain Relief

The muscles associated with arthritic joints are always likely to be tense, tight and painful. There are key features which help to maintain pain when muscles are tense and tight: an inadequate supply of fresh oxygenated blood, and retention/congestion/build-up of waste products in the tissues.

Massage can very successfully help to normalize both these features, even if only for a short time.

Massage also produces relaxation and a reduction in anxiety levels (especially when skilfully performed). To some extent, self-massage can achieve this too.

Self-massage or massage performed by a partner or family member can be very effective if it involves application of *rhythmic* strokes to the muscles in a systematic manner – although nothing can compare with the treatment of a professionally trained massage therapist.

Contraindications: Do not give yourself or anyone else a massage if the contraindications listed below exist:

- Avoid tissues which are actively inflamed or where blood vessels are inflamed.
- Avoid massaging where active infection is present.
- Avoid massaging if there is a heart condition unless professional advice supports doing so.
- Avoid massage if there is a cancerous condition – although there is evidence of benefit in such cases,

the massage has to be done under professional guidance.

- Avoid massage if there has been haemorrhage or other causes of bleeding in the tissues.
- Do not massage in the area of a recent fracture or sprain.

Basic Techniques
The following techniques are easily learned for use at home – massage should never hurt and should be performed slowly and rhythmically.

Effleurage
A massage cream or oil should be applied to the skin over the area to be massaged so that no 'drag' occurs on the skin.

The first movements call for slow, long strokes using the heel of the hands, the palm of the hands or the thumbs. The hands should be relaxed but firm and should mould themselves to the shape and contours of the area being worked on.

No pain should be produced and the pressure should match the sensitivity of the area.

Ideally, as one hand is moving forwards over the area (in the direction of the heart) the other should be coming back so that an alternating, rhythmic series of pleasant stroking actions soothes the region. Often a circular action is appropriate, so that one hand is following the other in slow, pleasing circles.

On a large area such as the thigh, make a stroke away from you with the heel of the hand for about 12 inches (30 cm) and then circle back again. As the hand is slowly returning towards you, the other commences its stroke. You are now doing effleurage!

Continue with this sort of approach for several minutes, varying the area slightly after a few repetitions. Use a similar pattern again after some of the other methods described below, and perhaps finish the whole session with stroking as well.

As suggested above, there is a convention which suggests that effleurage should usually be performed with the stroke moving towards the heart (up the leg, for example). This is not always easy when massaging parts of yourself, however; perhaps more important are the guidelines not to cause pain and to try to get a feeling of relaxation of the tissues.

Petrissage

This action is a kneading, wringing one in which muscles are held and lifted by one hand and then the other. One hand grasps a handful of muscle firmly but gently, lifting and pulling it towards you while the other pushes the adjacent tissue away from you, producing a kneading, squeezing and wringing action.

Start by pressing downwards with the heel of one hand while you lift the tissue with the fingers and thumb of that hand. With a handful of muscle, lift and gently squeeze or roll it before letting the other hand take over the same task. Repeat this process, one hand releasing its grip as the other takes over (just like making bread), several times rhythmically before moving to another part of the muscle.

In some areas two hands can work simultaneously lifting, wringing and twisting the tissues.

Tapping

Tapping and vibration of tissues can be very relaxing and can reduce pain sensations markedly. Try shaking the tissues gently, getting a vibration effect, or use the side of your hand to make a series of chopping actions towards the muscle so that the fingertips (relaxed) strike the muscle like drumsticks hitting a drum. By doing this lightly, quickly and repetitively a very pleasing sensation can be created.

Thumb Work

Wherever you feel local tension in the muscles or bands of tight tense tissue, use the thumbs or heel of your hand to push across or into the area, never to cause pain but sufficiently hard to produce a 'nice hurt'. Hold such pressure for up to 10 seconds at a time before moving on or applying a gentle effleurage to soothe it.

Tennis Ball Massage

Some areas are hard to reach, such as the low back, and you may need help to massage here.

Place a tennis ball on the carpet and lie on it so that it presses in the area of muscular pain. Gently roll over it so that it presses and pushes the muscle until you feel easier.

A similar effect can be achieved for the sole of the foot using a squash or golf ball.

Hydrotherapy Methods

Hydrotherapy can also be used safely to help in rheumatic and arthritic joints. It is important to realize that, in certain conditions, cold is infinitely more desirable than heat. The main reason for avoiding cold is that, in some individuals, there is inadequate vitality to respond to such a stimulus. If anyone is febrile, and very weak, then cold applications are best avoided, until the general state of health has improved adequately to respond positively. As a general rule, hot applications or alternate hot and cold applications, are better suited to long-standing, chronic conditions. Cold applications are better suited to active inflammatory conditions.

Hydrotherapy can be applied locally or generally, and the following methods are recommended for either osteoarthritis or rheumatoid arthritis.

Cold Compress

The cold compress is ideal for all inflamed or stiff joints. Despite its name it is designed to bring warmth to the area. It is applied cold, but is covered and insulated so as to allow body heat to warm it. A piece of cotton material, large enough to cover the area (wrist, knee, etc.) is wrung out in cold tap water, so that it is just damp, but not dripping wet. If the patient is not unduly affected by cold, and has good vitality and circulation, then two thicknesses of material should be used. Patients with poor circulation should settle for one thickness. The compress is placed over the joint and is immediately covered by one or two thicknesses of a flannel or woollen material, which is firmly safety-pinned in place. This is left in position for between 4 and 8 hours, unless it fails to warm up within 10 to 15 minutes. If after this period it still feels cold and clammy, then it was either too damp at the outset or was inadequately insulated. It should be removed and a further attempt made the next day. Normally it should gradually warm up and will be dry by the time it is removed. It can be left on overnight. The compress has a beneficial effect on the local circulation, as well as on the muscles overlying the joint. It will reduce pain and leave the area feeling easier and more pliable. The cold compress can be used on alternate days. The material used should be well washed after each use, as acid wastes are absorbed from the skin.

Alternate Hot and Cold Bathing

This method is ideal for either acute or chronic joints which are stiff, painful, swollen or inflamed. In order to stimulate the local circulation and reduce swelling and inflammation in an arthritic joint, the use of contrast bathing is ideal. This can be done in a number of ways, depending upon the joints involved. A small joint such as a finger or wrist can be treated under hot and cold running water, or in two bowls with water of appropriate temperatures. The hot water should be of such a temperature as to feel sufficiently hot, but without scalding the skin. The cold water should be very cold. Running tap water is ideal, but if a bowl is used ice should be floated in the cold water to maintain the temperature. The timing of the alternations is important. The hot treatment should last not less than 10 seconds, and the cold not less than 5 seconds, alternating 10 to 15 times and finishing with a cold treatment. If a joint is not suitable for either of the methods mentioned (e.g. hip), towels should be dipped in hot or cold water, lightly wrung out and then placed over or round the affected area. The timing is much the same, so that the towel remains in position for just long enough to prepare the contrasting one. It is a good idea to move and stretch the affected joint gently during and after the hydrotherapy treatment.

Epsom Salt Bathing

This method is ideal for rheumatic-arthritic conditions and can be used for the whole body, or a local joint. However, it is more suitable for chronic stiff conditions than acute inflamed ones. If whole-body Epsom salt bathing is undertaken the patient must be of reasonably sound disposition, as it is a little energy-draining. It is a marvellous method for helping to eliminate toxic wastes via the skin, and is very relaxing. Place, in a normal bath, approximately 2 lb of commercial Epsom salt (available from any chemist), $^1/_2$ lb of common salt (ideally sea salt) and a dessertspoon of iodine. The bath should be at a temperature of 100–104°F/ 37.7–40°C and the patient should spend between 10 and 20 minutes immersed in the water, which should be periodically topped up to maintain the heat. After the bath the patient should be briskly rubbed down, placed in a warm bed and well covered. Normally perspiration is induced by the bath, even in individuals who perspire infrequently. The patient should be given some hours to regain a normal body temperature before venturing out of bed. The Epsom salt bath should be not used more than once a week, as it is tiring.

A local joint can be treated in a similar fashion, by soaking it in hot water containing Epsom salt, salt and iodine. A hand, foot or elbow can be rested in hot water of this sort for 5 to 10 minutes, then wrapped in flannel after gentle stretching exercises. The area can be moved and stretched during the bathing as well as afterwards. If an area is too large to 'dunk' in this way, then a towel soaked in the water and wrung out so that it is just damp can be placed over the area. This should be replaced at frequent intervals to maintain the heat.

General Exercise in Water

As mentioned in the discussion on general exercise, swimming offers the opportunity to move and stretch joints in a weight-free environment. There are a number of heated pools available in most towns and cities. Some are attached to hospitals, some are private and some belong to local authorities. In an uncrowded, heated pool, it should be possible to undertake regular exercise and thereby to tone weak muscles, stretch tight joints and lessen the aggravation of sensitive, inflamed tissues. Information regarding hydrotherapy facilities can be obtained from local health authorities or Citizens Advice Bureaux.

Cryotherapy

As mentioned in the section dealing with trigger points, it is possible to use ice or cold sprays on inflamed areas to advantage. This should be done in such a way as to avoid frosting the skin or causing any deep cold ache. By chilling the tissues over and around a joint, and then stretching the tissues by slow movement, improved movement can be achieved and pain reduced. If the patient's vitality and circulation are very poor these methods may not be advisable.

One of the easiest methods is to take a large bag of frozen peas, wrap it in a tea towel and place it against a painful joint or muscle. After 5 to 10 minutes move the area gently and do not re-apply the cold bag for at least another hour.

There are many other methods of hydrotherapy, but the above are the safest and most desirable for the rheumatic-arthritic conditions under consideration.

Skin Friction Methods

The skin is a remarkable organ of elimination and we can greatly assist it in this function by regular use of skin friction methods. These are of value for all forms of rheumatic condition as long as they are carried out regularly and not too violently. Not only do they accelerate the removal of wastes from the skin, but they also enhance the lymphatic drainage of the body tissues.

The lymphatic system is a waste disposal system, via which a good deal of the breakdown products of life in the cells is carried away for ultimate detoxification and elimination from the body. With age and inactivity these channels become clogged to a large extent. This is especially true of anyone who is less active than usual because of arthritic changes. Skin friction or skin brushing has a remarkable effect on the lymphatic flow, helping to reduce swelling in joints. The methods have been in use for many years and are a major part of the revitalizing processes employed by leading health spas.

The method could not be simpler and involves the use of a brush made with natural (not plastic) bristles, a glove made of hemp or a loofah. Most major chemist chains will stock one or other of these. The brush, glove or loofah is kept dry. The best time for carrying out the (almost) daily ritual is first thing in the morning.

As much of the body surface as is reachable should be brushed (apart from the face). Start if possible with the skin on the feet, both underneath and on top. Then, with light strokes at first, sweep up the legs, front and back, to the buttocks and hips. The degree of firmness depends upon sensitivity; with regular use this will become greater, but at first it will be light. When the abdomen is reached the strokes should be gentle as the skin is much more sensitive here, and a circular motion should be used, going from the top right side of the abdomen across to the left, down and across to the right and then up again to the starting point. This clockwise motion follows the pattern of digestive peristalsis and is conducive to bowel health. Brush up to the chest and neck and over the shoulders, up the arms and as much of the back as you can manage, continuing firmly but gently to brush and stimulate the skin.

If areas are particularly swollen or sensitive due to arthritis, then avoid direct brushing over these. If restriction of movement is such as to make the procedures difficult, then a family member or friend can do this for you.

Ideally skin brushing should be followed by a shower or a bath. The tingling sense of well-being which will be felt is worth the effort. The benefits to the arthritic are of speedier elimination of acid wastes and a far healthier degree of internal drainage. It is suggested that this be done five or six days a week, or every day for three weeks, and then leaving a week free. The break somehow allows the degree of response to remain high, whereas constant use eventually produces a slowing down of this desirable reaction.

Aromatherapy

The selection of oils described below have proven herbal properties for stress-reduction, pain relief and sleep enhancement – *none is meant to be consumed.*

* When being added to a bath, the oils are used neat in the running water, which disperses and mixes them. If used for massage they should be combined with a neutral carrier oil (from any chemist).

- Store essential oils, individually or in combinations, in clean glass containers (dark if possible) away from light, tightly capped.

The various indications given below for each oil, and combinations of oils, can help you to select the one(s) most useful for your present state of health.

Basil

Basil has antiseptic properties as well as being an anti-depressant and a tonic for the digestion.

It can be used on its own (20 drops in the bath) to treat weakness, fatigue (including mental tiredness/fogginess) headaches, nausea, feelings of tension or faintness and depression.

Chamomile

Chamomile soothes, enhances sleep, acts as a digestive and general tonic, provides pain-relief and is an anti-bacterial agent.

It can be used on its own (20 drops in the bath) to treat sleep and digestive disturbances, skin conditions, neuralgia and inflammation. It soothes tired and irritated eyes when used as a compress or eyewash.

Combined with sage (10 drops of each in the bath) it helps with menopausal symptoms.

Cypress

This is an astringent, antispasmodic and tonic, and is useful as a deodorant.

It can be used alone (20 drops in the bath) to treat rheumatic and muscular conditions, coughs, flu and nervous tension.

Combined with lavender – 20 drops of each in warm water – it is useful for menopausal problems or for general nervous system treatment.

Lavender

This is an antispasmodic, antiseptic and general 'restorative'. Used alone (20 drops in the bath) it can help to alleviate stress and treat nervous problems or headache.

With cypress (as above) it eases menopausal or 'nervous system' problems. With vetiver (10 drops of each) it is helpful for anxiety.

Neroli

This is an antidepressant, antiseptic and digestive aid, as well as being said to be both a sedative and aphrodisiac.

Use by itself (20 drops in the bath) to treat depression, insomnia and nervous tension, digestive upsets and lack of sexual interest.

Use with basil (10 drops of each) in cases of anxiety, tension or depression.

Also – rosemary and/or eucalyptus can be added to any of the combinations above for specific effects on rheumatic and arthritic conditions.

Shock Absorbers in the Shoes

The use of shock-absorbing insoles in shoes has been proved to produce up to 50 per cent reduction in pain and stiffness in people suffering with arthritic changes in the pelvis and low back, by the simple means of reducing the stress passing through these regions. It is suggested therefore that anyone thus afflicted should ensure they wear cushioned soles or insoles. One simple method is to buy jogging shoes, which are superbly cushioned, and to use these for everyday walking around the home and garden. A good shoe shop will advise on alternative methods of improving cushioning in shoes.

We have considered general body mechanics and exercise as well as relaxation methods in the relief of pain and stiffness. Obviously, these methods all deal with existing states of dysfunction in joints, and so presume a degree of existing stiffness and disability. In order to reverse the potential worsening of this condition it is also vital that we consider the biochemistry of the body. This means that we must consider nutrition in our search for safe self-help methods.

4
Arthritis and Nutrition

Probably no aspect of life has such a dramatic influence on health generally, and on arthritis (in all its forms) in particular, as what we eat. There are a number of specific nutrients which, when in short supply, have been found to influence arthritis adversely. These can greatly assist in checking and sometimes overcoming the symptoms of arthritis. Additionally, there are foods which irritate and aggravate arthritis. These can include either highly acidic foods, or foods to which the individual is 'sensitive' or allergic.

General Strategy to Reduce Inflammation

Irrespective of the cause of inflammation, there are several anti-inflammatory nutritional methods which are useful in most pain and arthritis situations.

Inflammation is a natural and mostly useful response by the body to irritation, injury and infection. It can be a major part of the process of getting better, despite the fact that it is not exactly pleasant. Therefore, altering or reducing inflammation drastically may be counterproductive. If nutritional tactics of inflammation reduction are used, they should be first discussed with a health care professional and agreed that they represent a safe way forward.

If pain is reduced by these methods, or any others, it is a mistake to use this as a licence to become very active, if this will lead to stress on a previously inflamed or damaged area. Remember that overuse of damaged areas (joint surfaces) is one of the reasons why arthritic joints get worse when the pain is eased by drugs.

So use nutritional anti-inflammatory pain-relieving methods with respect and under advice if the pain is of long standing or from a cause which you do not understand, and don't over-do activity when pain eases. It is always safer to have professional advice rather than hoping for the best in such matters.

Dietary Tactics

Reduce Animal Fats

A major part of the pain/inflammation process involves minute chemical substances which your body makes, called prostaglandins and leukotrienes. These are themselves to a great extent dependent upon the presence of arachidonic acid, which humans manufacture mainly from animal fats. This means that reducing your animal fat intake cuts down your access to the enzymes which help to produce arachidonic acid, and therefore cuts down the levels of the inflammatory substances released in tissues which contribute so greatly to pain. Cutting down or eliminating animal fats is then the first priority in an anti-inflammatory dietary approach.

- Fat-free or low-fat milk, yogurt and cheese should be eaten in preference to full-fat varieties, and butter avoided altogether.
- Meat fat should be completely avoided, and since much fat in meat is invisible, meat itself can be left out of the diet for a time (or permanently). Poultry skin should also be avoided.
- 'Hidden' fats in products such as biscuits and other manufactured foods should be avoided – always check product labels.

Eat More Fish

Fish and taking fish oil are OK: Some fish, mainly those which come from cold water areas such as the North sea, contain high levels of eicosapentenoic acid (EPA), which reduces levels of arachidonic acid in tissues and therefore helps to create fewer inflammatory substances in the body. Most importantly, fish oil has these anti-inflammatory effects without interfering with the useful jobs which some prostaglandins do, such as protection of the delicate stomach lining and maintaining the correct level of blood clotting. This is important because there are many drugs which can do just what fish oil does (reducing inflammation and therefore pain) but unfortunately only by also causing new problems, something EPA does not do (unless you happen to be allergic to fish).

Research has shown that using EPA in rheumatic and arthritic conditions offers relief from swelling, stiffness and pain, although benefits do not usually become evident until fish oil supplements have been taken for 3 months, reaching their most effective level after around 6 months.

If you want to follow this strategy:

- Eat fish such as herring, sardine, salmon and mackerel at least twice weekly (more often if you wish).
- Take EPA capsules (10 to 15 daily) when inflammation is at its worst, until relief appears, and then a maintenance dose of 6 daily.

EPA and Arthritis

Some years ago, the American Dr Dong concluded after treating his own arthritic condition that the approach which achieved the best results involved the elimination from the diet of dairy products and saturated fats. This was before knowledge of free radicals (see page 90) was widespread, and indicates that he had found, by trial and error, a method of reducing substances in the body which are readily oxidized – that is, animal fats. The eating of proteins such as fish and chicken was encouraged on Dr Dong's diet, as was the abundant use of vegetables.

This is a simplification of the diet which he recommended, but is of particular interest since a study subsequently published in the *Lancet* indicated that by reducing saturated fats from the diet (i.e. no dairy products and no red meat) and increasing the sources of polyunsaturated fats (vegetable origin) and EPA, there was a marked improvement in the condition of rheumatoid arthritics.

It was found in medical trials that the group of rheumatoid arthritic patients who followed this type of dietary regime achieved markedly less swollen and less painful joints and less morning stiffness (a characteristic of rheumatoid arthritis) than did the control group of patients who took a dummy supplement. It is important to realize that the improvements noted were not clearly evident until after 12 weeks of following the diet. The researchers pointed out that: 'Changes in tissue lipids (fats) are not seen until six weeks after a change in diet.'

When the participants in the study were re-examined some months after the trial, the group of patients who had had the EPA supplements had deteriorated rapidly (within 2 weeks of stopping the supplements), indicating that the programme needs to be continued indefinitely if progress is to be maintained. This is an important injunction for anyone with a long-term arthritic condition: Once improvement is noted it is most unwise to abandon the pattern of diet and nutrients being followed, as a return of symptoms is likely.

These methods are seldom able to approach the true causes of the condition in rheumatoid arthritis – which, as indicated, remain a mystery. They do, however, provide a strategy by which control can be achieved safely, in many cases.

EPA is available in capsules of around 300 mg. The suggested dose is 1,800 mg daily (6 capsules per day), taken in 3, 2-capsule doses throughout the day. Red meat was allowed in the medical trials only twice per week, and then only if lean cuts were used with visible fat removed. Dr Dong, however, suggested in his findings that it be permanently abandoned. Chicken was allowed if the skin was avoided. Sausage, bacon and all lunch meats were banned, as was whole milk, cheese and saturated cooking oils (lard, butter, hydrogen-saturated shortenings and margarine).

Anyone attempting this diet should eat an abundance of vegetables and wholegrain cereal products (see page 80 for discussion of the allergy-arthritis link), and avoid white flour products and all sugar if possible. Alcohol should also be avoided.

Deficiencies

We are all genetically unique and this has been shown to result in individuals having idiosyncratic requirements for particular nutrients. Certain people need far more of some particular nutrients than others, and this requirement manifests itself in a particular pattern of symptoms. The requirement may be for any of the nutrients (e.g. minerals, vitamins, amino acids) which the body requires for normal functioning. In regard to arthritis we would normally be concerned with a particular group of nutrients involved with the integrity of the ligaments, tendons, cartilaginous tissue, muscles and bones. We will now examine each of these groups.

Minerals

Calcium
This is the mineral which is most useful for improving the tone and elasticity of the soft tissues around the joints. Calcium also assists in the transportation of nerve impulses from one part of the body to another. This function is directly involved with another aspect of

the work of calcium, which is in promoting the efficient contraction and relaxation of muscles. Normally, over 90 per cent of calcium which is ingested is incorporated into the body structures, with the rest being involved in other functions, including those mentioned above. Surveys in the US indicate that over 30 per cent of the population is calcium deficient. With inadequate calcium, muscles cannot contract adequately. This can lead to joint instability. Also, if calcium is lacking there is a 'softening' of bone, which can lead to overprotective spasms in the soft tissues supporting these bones, and consequent stiffness and pain. In such circumstances, simply taking calcium is unlikely to be effective, since it interacts with other nutrients. Extra zinc and magnesium are also necessary to correct calcium deficiency.

Magnesium

This nutrient is often called 'nature's tranquillizer'. It enhances the body's ability to contract muscles. The symptoms of magnesium deficiency include muscle tremors as well as loss of calcium and potassium, leading to cramps. Since the processing of food often results in magnesium being eliminated, there is widespread deficiency in modern society. It is vital that calcium and magnesium are supplemented together, preferably in a ratio of two parts calcium to one part magnesium.

Manganese

This is a vital component of enzymes involved with the musculo-skeletal system. Manganese deficiency is evident when collagen (the supporting soft tissue material) is not functioning normally. It has been said by experts in physical therapy that supplementation of manganese doubles the success rate of the treatment of joint problems.

Zinc

This most important mineral is vitally linked with the healing of irritated tissues. It is also involved in calcium metabolism. In treating rheumatoid arthritis, Dr Carl Pfeiffer of the famous Brain-Bio Center in the US has used zinc with great success. He points out that arthritic sufferers usually show a high copper level in the body. He believes that zinc drives copper from the inflamed joint. When copper is in excess and zinc is being used to counter this, the amino acid l-histidine has been used successfully in doses of between 1 and 6 grams a day to help normalize the biochemistry of the inflamed joints. Zinc is used at Pfeiffer's Center in doses of 200 mg a day, until improvement is noted (for up to 12 weeks). The only side-effect noted was mild diarrhoea. Zinc also has a beneficial effect on the defence mechanism of the body. Vitamin B_6 is employed at the same time as zinc therapy, as both are closely associated in their work.

All minerals mentioned in this chapter are best taken as 'chelates'. This means that they are linked with easily absorbed proteins which enables better uptake and utilization by the body.

Vitamins

Vitamin B complex

The vitamin B complex has special importance to the functioning of the nervous system. It is involved in the stability of nerve structures and function, as well as the musculo-skeletal system. Muscle tone is particularly influenced by vitamin B_1 (thiamin), which also helps in the elimination of toxic wastes. Vitamin B_3 (niacin) has been shown to stimulate local circulation, improve joint mobility, decrease stiffness and bring relief to many distorted and painful joints. Dr William Kauffman of Stratford, Connecticut, first used B_3 for treating arthritis, and found it often helped. A trial in Sweden has also shown it to be effective, and also well-tolerated. Limitation of movement often responds dramatically to B_3. Vitamin B_5 (pantothenic acid or calcium pantothenate) has also been used to help the arthritic condition, by virtue of its effects on the adrenal gland, which defends us against stress. Many arthritic sufferers have been shown to be deficient in B_5.

Vitamin C

This vitamin takes part in many body processes. The health of bones, tendons, cartilages and connective tissues depends upon its presence in adequate amounts. Its major function from our viewpoint is that it is involved in the synthesis of collagen. This is a protein fibre found throughout the body's soft tissues, and is the body's main supporting tissue. It strengthens the 'cement' of the body, giving it integrity and stability. When vitamin C is deficient all body tissues are affected. Muscles weaken and ligaments grow so weak that they cannot support the joints.

Vitamin D

This is vital for the adequate uptake and utilization of calcium.

The nutrients discussed above are the most critical ones of which the arthritic sufferer should be aware. It is of course possible to obtain all these from a well-balanced diet, such as the one outlined later in this chapter. However, modern farming and processing methods may produce foods without enough of some of these substances to correct existing deficiencies. Therefore some short-term supplementation of calcium, magnesium, manganese, zinc, and vitamins C, D, B_1, B_3, B_5, and B_6 is often beneficial.

These supplements should be taken for at least 3 but preferably 6 months, before reviewing the situation; however, if symptoms are well under control then intake should be reduced or stopped.

Other Nutrients – Including Amino Acids and Enzymes

A potent and safe pain-reducing agent is an amino acid called phenylalanine. This occurs usually in the l-form, but there is also what is known as a 'right-handed', or d-form. This reduces the degradation of the body's own painkillers, the endorphins, and thus helps in the easing of pain.

The combination of d- and l-phenylalanine is known as DLPA, and is available from health food stores. By taking 2, 375-mg tablets about half an hour prior to meals 3 times a day for several weeks, pain of most sorts will diminish to tolerable levels, or will disappear altogether.

If after that period pain has not gone, then the dosage can be doubled for a further 2 weeks or so. If, in rare cases, there is still no improvement, then the method should be abandoned. In most cases there is improvement within a week, and at that point the tablets should be stopped, unless there is a recurrence (after some weeks or months). It must be remembered, however, that even if the pain goes the underlying condition remains unaltered, and the joints should not be overused. Pain can also be alleviated by taking vitamin B_3 (niacin). Check with a qualified nutritionist or health care provider for the current recommended dosage.

Glucosamine for Arthritis

Glucosamine is a substance which has incredible potential in treating conditions where conventional and alternative approaches have brought only relief, not cure.

On the basis of clinical data now available, glucosamine supplementation has been found to be extremely useful in the treatment of several disorders involving tissue injuries and joint inflammation.

Tissues inside and around the joints become damaged due to lack of efficient lubricating synovial fluids in the joint spaces. Instead of being thick and elastic, normal cushioning is impaired or lost altogether and, consequently, the bones and the lining cartilages chafe together inside the joint space. A loss of cushioning by watery bursae allows tendons to rub against the hard edges of bones. Cartilage starts to erode and problems arise, often involving arthritic changes.

In the spinal column, the individual vertebrae are stacked one on top of the other, separated only by the cushioning intervertebral discs. In the middle of each disc lies a cartilage that separates the vertebrae. This is crucial because many nerves exit from the spinal cord, and they do so through the spaces between the vertebrae. With injuries to these discs, the gelatinous cartilage becomes softer. As a result, the vertebrae move closer together and compress the nerves.

Glucosamine helps to restore the thick, gelatinous nature of the fluids and tissues in and around the joints, and in between the vertebrae. N-Acetyl Glucosamine and Glucosamine Sulphate are among the types of biological chemicals that form hyaluronic acid, a major cushioning ingredient of the joint fluids and surrounding tissues.

Normally we form enough Glucosamine Sulphate ourselves, but poor posture, stress, sports, ageing and free radical reactions rapidly deplete the body's natural supply. Glucosamine Sulphate supplementation can help to replenish levels in the body.

Glucosamine may give improvement in symptoms relating to:

- degeneration, swelling and inflammation of the synovial fluids
- osteoarthritis
- during recovery from joint injuries
- following operations and during recuperation
- damage to and inflammation of muscles
- slipped disc and sciatica
- dystrophy of joints associated with ageing
- injury and loss of elasticity of intervertebral disc.

Dosage suggestions: One tablet containing 400 mg Glucosamine Sulphate, 3 times a day for 1 month, then 1 tablet twice a day for the following month.

For optimal response, it is recommended that the Glucosamine be taken in conjunction with a good antioxidant complex containing vitamins A, C, E and selenium.

Anti-inflammatory (Proteolytic) Enzymes

Enzymes are minute chemical substance which take part in or commence all chemical reactions in the body and so are vital for life itself.

Some are very involved in digestion, such as protease, a major element in our digestion of protein.

It has been found that use of other protein-digesting enzymes derived from plants have a gentle but substantial anti-inflammatory influence. These include bromelaine, which comes from the pineapple plant, and papain, from the papaya plant. Health food stores and pharmacists sell these. Around 2 to 3 grams of one or other (bromelaine is the more effective) should be taken over the course of the day (away from mealtimes or all they will do is help digest your food) as part of an anti-inflammatory, pain-relieving strategy.

(See the notes on cysteine, histidine and bromelaine in Chapter 5 for details of amino acids and enzymes which can be helpful in the inflammatory stages of osteoarthritis as well as rheumatoid arthritis.)

General Rules of Eating and Diet

1. Digestion begins in the mouth. Food should be eaten slowly and chewed thoroughly.
2. Avoid foods that are very hot or very cold.
3. Avoid drinking any liquid with meals, as this interferes with digestion (as does any liquid taken up to an hour after a main meal).
4. Choose simple meals, as these are easier to digest than those with complicated sauces or dressings. Avoid combinations of certain foods that produce indigestion, such as protein and carbohydrate (e.g. bread and cheese, or fish and chips).
5. Avoid fried and roasted foods, as these are difficult to digest.
6. Don't drink instant coffee! It has been found that instant coffee contains substances which block the receptor sites used by our natural painkilling endorphins, making pain seem more intense. Although only found to be true of instant coffee, this is not a recommendation to drink brewed coffee instead, but a suggestion that at least instant coffee should be avoided by people in pain.

In any rheumatic condition the following pattern of diet will lead to an overall reduction in pain and improved function, especially if accompanied by the other methods outlined in this book. As individual differences exist it is difficult to be specific about desirable eating patterns. Therefore the following suggestions focus on those foods which should be avoided.

Salt and salted food – Avoid completely and replace with moderate amounts of potassium chloride and herbs.

Meat – Use modest amounts of fish or free-range poultry, i.e. no more than 3 oz/150 g daily. In acute conditions this should also be abandoned in favour of vegetable protein (pulse and cereal combinations).

Dairy produce – Apart from a little (4 oz/200 g daily) live goat's milk yogurt, replace milk with soya milk, and cheese with tofu (soya curd).

White flour or white rice products – Replace with wholemeal, millet and brown rice.

Sugar – Avoid completely.

Tea, coffee, chocolate, cola drinks – Avoid, replacing them with herbal teas, dandelion coffee and fresh vegetable drinks, or yeast extracts (if low salt), or spring water.

Processed, pickled, smoked, preserved, tinned foods – Avoid vinegar, pepper, curry.

Frozen foods – Strictly limit these, especially commercially frozen foods.

Acid fruits – Strictly limit plums, berries, citrus, etc.

The diet should comprise at least 50 per cent raw food in the form of vegetables, sprouted seeds (leave these out of your diet if you have rheumatoid arthritis, however) seeds, nuts, wholegrains and some fruit. Breakfast should be seed (sunflower, pumpkin, linseed, etc.), nut, grain millet or oat flakes mixed together with some fresh or dried non-acid fruit. In sub-acute conditions a little live yogurt can be added. One main meal each day should be a mixed salad with seeds and wholemeal bread, a rice savoury or a jacket potato. For five days of the week, the other main meal should be a cooked vegetable with a protein savoury (either fish or chicken or, ideally, a combined cereal and pulse dish). On the other two days a second salad meal should be eaten. Drinks should be as indicated above.

This diet is designed to minimize the chances of a continued deficiency; as well, it should reduce the acidification and toxification of the body, which is so prevalent a factor in arthritic and rheumatic conditions. By combining the suggested supplementary intake with this diet the self-healing mechanisms of the body will be given the best possible chance to carry out their task of repair to damaged areas and organs.

Fasting

Fasting is useful in the body's detoxification. It is one of the oldest methods of healing. It is instinctive in sick animals and probably was in primitive humans, too. As well as having psychic and spiritual benefits, fasting can be useful in preventing disease, if carried out sensibly. It is often confused with starvation but, strictly, it is abstinence for a given time from solid food, and not from liquids. The last point is controversial. Some experts say fasting is most effective if only water is taken, whereas others, myself included, advocate the intake of fruit and vegetable juices. Some strange things may happen to the body during a fast and it is best to understand them before beginning one so that they do not cause anxiety; they are, after all, signs of rejuvenation.

Fasting often results in a furred tongue, 'sick' headache, bad breath, dark and often offensive urine, and sometimes unusual bowel movements. The degree and intensity of these signs of detoxification will vary greatly from person to person, often depending on the underlying health and vitality of the individual as well as on the type of fast being used. Surprisingly, hunger is often not noticed after the first day.

Fasting can be seen as the preparation for self-healing. It is not a cure for anything. It provides a chance to eliminate toxins which are preventing the body from healing itself. So it is important not to treat the initial signs of fasting, such as a 'sick' headache, with any drugs or potions that will suppress them. These initial discomforts will soon disappear. A short fast may not be long enough for all these things to happen, but by repetition the intensity of the symptoms of the first fast will diminish. In time, fasts may be enjoyed without marked symptoms, which is a sign of increased health.

If a chronic illness is involved, such as arthritis or an allergic or catarrhal condition, then there is a good case for daily enemas or, for those who prefer, a herbal laxative, before and after the fast. Breaking the fast correctly is also important. After any length of time without solid food there must be a gentle transition back to a full diet. It is also important that during a fast some exercise is taken; staying in bed is seldom necessary, but plenty of rest is. Therefore it is unwise to fast while carrying on normal work. It is also unwise to drive during a fast because dizziness may occur. Fresh air and rest are important, as is the avoidance of stress. This explains the popularity of health farms and spas, which offer a restful environment.

Three-day fasts, done over a weekend, are a good introduction; such a fast is set out below. A 3-day detoxification, every 4 to 6 weeks, over 6 or 12 months, will produce a dramatic improvement in health. Alternatively you might prefer to fast for one day each week. A light meal can be eaten midday on a Saturday, followed by juice on Saturday evening through to Sunday evening, with the fast being broken Sunday evening or Monday morning. Such a fast, lasting 24 to 36 hours every week or fortnight, will also be beneficial to health.

In all cases the aim of fasting is to rest the body from the constant onslaught of food. This principle can also be applied to everyday eating to make us feel more vital and lively. For instance, 'breakfast' implies that we have been for a period without food. This is true if the last meal of the previous day was at 6 p.m. and breakfast is at 7 or 8 a.m., but if we eat after 9 p.m. the night before then the digestive system will barely have finished coping with the evening meal before the next lot of food starts to arrive. Such a pattern of eating makes people sluggish and lethargic. By eating earlier in the evening, with no snacks later on, you can be livelier in the morning and have a rested digestive system, ready for the next day. Longer fasts should only be undertaken with the help of a qualified nutritionist.

Preparing for a Fast

The day before fasting, a herbal laxative such as psyllium seeds, or a broth made of flax seeds (linseed), or castor oil should be taken after the midday meal, which should itself be light (vegetarian for preference, such as a mixed salad or a vegetable soup). In the evening have a light fruit meal (pear, apple, grapes), or a vegetable broth (recipe follows). On rising the next day drink either chamomile or peppermint tea (unsweetened), a cup of vegetable broth, half a cup of spring water with half a cup of carrot juice, or warm or cold apple juice (diluted with water). A selection of one of these items, or bottled spring water, should be consumed at 2- to 3-hour intervals during the day, making sure that vegetable broth is consumed at least twice during the day (not less than 1 pint daily), and that the total daily liquid intake is not less than 2 litres and not more than 4 litres. If fresh vegetable juice is not obtainable, Biotta vegetable juice is available at most health food stores and is suitable for fasting as it contains no preservatives, other than lactic acid, and is guaranteed organically grown. Carrot and beetroot are the ideal juices.

Continue this pattern for the 2 or 3 days of the fast and finish on the evening of the final day by eating one of the following 'meals': puréed cooked apple or pear; puréed carrot, plus a little puréed vegetable soup; live, natural yogurt can be eaten with either of these choices. All food should be chewed thoroughly and slowly. The next morning eat yogurt and grated apple or fresh pear, and have a salad and jacket potato for lunch, continuing with a normal pattern of eating. (Processed foods, such as white flour and sugar products, should be avoided and the diet should consist of wholefood). If any of the above foods cause allergies they should, of course, be avoided. For this reason it is best to fast under some degree of supervision.

If possible, a herbal laxative or castor oil or a warm water enema should be used on the last evening of the fast. If the patient is chronically ill, then daily small water enemas should be used during the fast. Half a pint of water at body heat is recommended.

The hygiene of the bowel can be further improved by employing one or all of the following, both during the fast and for a week or so afterwards. Take a quarter teaspoonful of a high quality acidophilus/bifidus combination daily. These highly concentrated acidophilus products will enhance the flora of the bowel; dairy-free probiotics are suitable for people who are milk-sensitive. Also, stir a teaspoonful of fine green clay powder into a small glass of spring water and allow it to settle for an hour. Drink the water, but not the sediment. The clay has a detoxifying effect and soothes the bowel.

During the Fast

Expect to feel lethargic during the fast, and perhaps a degree colder; wear an extra layer of clothing. Rest as much as possible, since the aim is to allow energy to be employed towards healing, not diffused in unnecessary activity. Take no medication of any sort. In people of normal weight the fast will result in a number of predictable and beneficial effects, but it will not have the same physiological effects in very overweight individuals. One of these beneficial effects is the release of a growth hormone by the pituitary gland. This hormone has many functions, including fat mobilization. As individuals of normal weight release more of the hormone than overweight ones, the benefits are greater for them. A short fast by an overweight person is quite in order, provided that their general health is stable (and they do not suffer from diabetes, etc.). Fasting is safe if employed correctly, and is one of the swiftest detoxifying and health-promoting methods available. Try it regularly.

Making Your Own Vegetable Broth

If possible use organically-grown vegetables. If this is not possible then scrub vegetables well before use. Into 2 litres of spring water place 750 g/4 cupfuls of finely chopped beetroot, carrots, thick potato peelings, parsley, courgette and leaves of beetroot or parsnip. Use no sulphur-rich vegetables such as cabbage or onions, which might produce gas. Simmer for 5 minutes over a low flame, to allow the breakdown of vegetable fibre and the release of nutrients into the liquid. Cool and strain, using only the liquid and not the leftover vegetable content. Do not add salt, as this broth will contain ample natural minerals and will provide nutrients without straining the digestive system. Also, it is alkaline and neutralizes any acidity resulting from the fast. Drink at least 1 pint of this nutritious broth daily during the fast.

Allergy

One of the most important contributions to our knowledge of arthritic conditions has come from practitioners dealing with allergies. Many of these practitioners call themselves clinical ecologists, and they have shown that by the removal from the diet of foods which cause allergies, many arthritic conditions can be improved. In attempting to ascertain which foods produce allergies in patients, many practitioners use a period of fasting to clear the body of all toxic substances. They then reintroduce foods one at a time to gauge the body's reaction. In this way they can build a picture of undesirable foods which should be avoided. Sometimes, those foods which cause a reaction can be reintroduced by using a rotation diet. The allergy-producing foods may be consumed on infrequent occasions, say once a week. By eliminating dairy produce and refined carbohydrates (e.g. white flour and sugar) from the diet we remove some of the foods which most commonly cause allergies.

By employing short and regular fasts, and by using nutritional supplements, the likelihood is that food sensitivities or allergies will be further eliminated. However, it may be that a commonly eaten food continues to irritate the joints and this may show up after a fast when the particular food is reintroduced. If such a food is identified, then it should be used sparingly in the diet. It is also useful to identify other foods belonging to the same group as the one which causes the allergy. These should also be rotated, so that they are not used more than once in 5 days.

Self-testing for Sensitivities and Allergies
Expert advice and guidance is needed in dealing with food intolerances which are common in arthritic conditions. Many tests exist, none of them foolproof and some with a tendency to produce false-positive and false-negative results. The most accurate method is to test suspect foods by eliminating them (for at least 5 days), looking for a reduction in symptoms (or not) and then reintroducing the food and reassessing symptom patterns.

Pulse Test
A simple 'pulse test' is sometimes an accurate guide to food sensitivity. The pulse is taken before eating a particular food and then again at intervals after its ingestion – 20 minutes, 40, 60 and perhaps 120 minutes later. If the pulse rate changes by at least 10 beats per minute, either upwards or downwards, the food is suspect and should be avoided for at least a week before being retested. If the food is indeed provoking a reaction, then if it is eaten twice on a single day, following a week's exclusion, the pulse rate should rise or fall by at least 10 beats per minute some time after (sometimes

immediately following) a meal containing the suspect food, and symptoms such as fatigue, increased pain or palpitations might appear. The food should then be eliminated from the diet for at least 6 months.

Exclusion and Rotation Diets

In general, food allergy and intolerance is dealt with by eliminating the offending food through specific exclusion or hypoallergenic diets – such as a lamb and pear diet, or a monodiet (say rice only) – or a Stone age dietary pattern which eliminates all grains and dairy produce as well as modern processed foods, or by short-term (usually 5-day) fasting – followed by reintroduction of suspected foods to assess their impact on symptoms.

Rotation

Alternative methods include rotation diets in which suspect foods are eaten infrequently (no more than once in 5 days) to avoid sensitization or allergic responses. The various methods currently in use by clinical ecologists or allergy specialists all require patience, conscious dedicated application and sound advice to be effective.

Stress reduction is also vital in dealing with allergy/ sensitivity problems.

If bowel malabsorption problems exist, resulting perhaps from yeast or parasite activity, then the bowel condition needs to be sorted out concurrently or before the allergy is tackled.

Sometimes allergy happens when incomplete digestion of food occurs, due to inadequate hydrochloric acid levels or poor digestive enzyme production. Expert nutritional help can assist in normalizing these imbalances.

Food Intolerance

The foods most commonly causing sensitivity for all conditions are wheat, corn, yeast, milk, eggs, fish, shellfish, citrus fruits, chocolate, tomatoes (nightshade family), strawberries and nuts.

The most accurate and least expensive way by means of which you can discover an intolerance/sensitivity is to follow an elimination diet and test the suspected foods one by one.

The elimination diet will give highly effective results with no serious side-effects and little, if any, expense.

About 5 days are needed to clear the bowel completely of foods that were eaten before the diet was begun. By this time, most people will be relieved of problems caused by their food sensitivities. Another week is then needed before you test the suspect foods.

Step-by-step Procedure for Testing

1. Be sure to eat the test foods regularly prior to the elimination diet: make sure you eat the test foods at

least once on each of 3 successive days prior to the beginning of the elimination diet. This is most important for the testing to be successful.

2. Diary: keep a careful diary of everything you eat beginning 3 days prior to the beginning of the diet until the testing is ended.

3. Elimination diet: you will be on the elimination diet for about 2 weeks. Even one little bite of a 'forbidden' food will distort the results. Make no other additions, changes or substitutions in the diet.

4. During the elimination diet you may feel worse on the second or third day. These withdrawal symptoms are not uncommon and may be relieved by taking 2 tablets of Alka-Seltzer Gold.

5. After 2 weeks of elimination of the food being tested, all the while eating normally and keeping a symptom 'score sheet', reintroduce the food on a daily basis for at least 3 days to evaluate whether symptoms are aggravated.

6. Test foods: Leave each of these out of your diet – one at a time – for 2 weeks. If after this time there has been an improvement, reintroduce the food and monitor the effects. If there is no benefit from exclusion, simply reintroduce and go on to the next exclusion test.

Dairy – milk, cheese, butter (replace with rice milk, soya milk or oat milk)

Yeast-based foods (including mushrooms and bread made with yeast – you can get unyeasted 'sourdough' or soda bread instead for this trial period, as well as rice cakes, Ryvita biscuits, etc. Read labels carefully during this exclusion period)

Wheat in all its forms – a difficult task but worth the effort! Replace with pure rye bread (be sure of this, as most 'rye bread' contains wheat) or rice cakes, or Ryvita biscuits

Nightshade family (tomato, potato, aubergine, pepper)

Citrus fruits

Corn

any other foods you commonly eat.

If you feel better when you exclude a food and worse when you reintroduce it, then leave it out of your diet for at least 6 months before testing it again.

In general, a combination of all the factors discussed above, namely diet, detoxification, exclusion of foods to which your body is intolerant, and replenishment of nutrient deficiencies, provides a framework for alleviating arthritic conditions of all sorts. In addition, exercise and hydrotherapy are beneficial.

5
Rheumatoid Arthritis

The causes of rheumatoid arthritis are not fully understood. Although the minutiae of the actual changes involved in the arthritic process are well documented, the causes remain largely a matter for speculation. One cause, which applies in some cases only, involves the presence in the arthritic joint of virus particles. This has led to a line of enquiry which points to some common childhood ailments as being a possible starting point, and also to immunization against these conditions being implicated.

Rubella Vaccination and Juvenile (and Adult) Arthritis

One condition in particular has a history of producing juvenile arthritis and that is Rubella (German Measles) and vaccination against this. German measles is not a particularly serious problem for children, but vaccination is performed in order to protect the female population so that they do not contract the disease when they are of childbearing age and thereby risk having malformed babies. Males are immunized in the hope that this will reduce the general level of the infection in society, in order ultimately to wipe it out.

All this is laudable in its intention, if debatable as to its efficacy. Unfortunately one of the commonest side-effects of rubella vaccination is arthritis and polyneuralgia. Much of this is transient and leaves no permanent damage. However, there is evidence of wider damage in many young bodies.

How Widespread Is This?

The following report has been published in *Science* magazine: 'The HEW [US Department of Health, Education and Welfare] reported in 1970 that as much as 26 per cent of children (over 1 in 4) receiving rubella vaccination developed arthralgia or arthritis. Many had to seek medical attention, and some were hospitalized.'

Adults too are vaccinated against this, since young women who did not contract the illness in childhood and who are anticipating parenthood might well be persuaded as to its desirability.

In Canada it is reported (Humanitarian Society, Quakertown, Pennsylvania 1983) that 30 per cent of adults given rubella vaccine suffered arthritis attacks within 4 weeks, some of these of crippling intensity. Dr Glenn Dettman of Australia reports that live rubella viruses have been found in one third of children and adults suffering rheumatoid arthritis.

In October 1985, the *New England Journal of Medicine* reported: 'Infection, or immunization with rubella virus, has been recognized as producing acute synovitis (inflammation of joint capsules) which although usually self-limiting has been reported to recur for months or years after the acute stage.' The report continues by stating that a full 35 per cent of people suffering chronic joint disease (such as juvenile rheumatoid arthritis, spondyloarthritis and polyarticular rheumatoid arthritis) were carrying rubella virus particles. These were never found in people who did not have joint diseases.

It seems likely, therefore, that a large proportion of rheumatoid arthritis is, partly or totally, the result of immunization techniques. Another major cause of rheumatoid arthritis, which is partially understood, involves what is called autoimmune processes. This means that an allergic reaction is underway, and the tissues which are being reacted against as 'foreign' to the body are its own joints and soft tissues. Thus the body is literally appearing to want to eliminate or destroy its own tissues. Being allergic to oneself is not a pleasant prospect, and understanding just how this might have occurred requires awareness of the immune system, the body's defence mechanisms, and health.

One major aspect of immune function is related to the thymus gland, which lies within the chest. The thymus is responsible for mobilizing the white blood cells of the body into action against any possible invading micro-organisms or foreign protein (cancer cells, malabsorbed foods, etc.). The cells which it calls up in a crisis are called T-cells (T for thymus). These in turn produce substances called lymphokines which are natural defenders of the body (one of these is called interferon, a potent anti-cancer weapon produced by the T-cells).

The T-cells also produce macrophages which literally 'eat up' or engulf bacteria, cancer cells, etc. Part of the T-cell function is to balance against the overzealous action of other defending white blood cells, called B-cells, which produce antibodies against any invading substances or bacteria. If there are too few T-cells, then the B-cells can be so active that they destroy the very tissues of the body. The T-cells are suppressors of over-enthusiastic B-cell function, and so the balance between these different 'soldiers' of the body is a vital part in maintaining health.

When autoimmune disease is operating, such as in rheumatoid arthritis, cancer, ulcerative colitis, multiple sclerosis and diabetes, B-cells are predominant and

T-cells in short supply. Part of any strategy to improve such a condition should therefore involve an attempt to rebalance this situation, and to assist thymus activity and consequent T-cell activity. The mineral and vitamin support recommended in this and previous chapters will enhance T-cell function considerably. The nutrients most valuable in this task are also strong antioxidants (see below) which makes them doubly useful. They include vitamins C and E, as well as a number of the B complex vitamins (notably B_6, B_5 [pantothenic acid], and folic acid) as well as zinc and selenium.

Free Radicals and Arthritis

When metal is exposed to oxygen for too long it oxidizes, or rusts. When an apple or potato is peeled, it changes colour rapidly as it oxidizes. When hair is bleached with hydrogen peroxide it changes colour, as this powerful oxidant destroys the pigment (and something of the structure) of the hair. As we get older our tissues, such as skin, show signs of ageing, and wrinkling becomes apparent; this too is largely a process of oxidation.

All of these examples involve the presence of substances called free radical oxidizers, highly active elements which, because of their structure, are able to disrupt other cells by 'stealing' atoms from them, which alters their structure. A wide variety of changes ensue and it is not within the scope of this book to explore these fully, apart from pointing to the fact that many inflammatory processes involve a virtually uncontrolled series of free radical chemical changes.

It is a part of the normal body defence mechanism to produce free radicals, a process by which blood cells destroy invading enemies. If the body produces its own free radical, and with it destroys an invading micro-organism, for example, then it relies upon the presence in the body of antioxidants to 'quench' the process when it has usefully done its job.

There are, within the healthy body, a large number of free radical deactivators, or scavengers, which mop up surplus oxidative elements such as this, preventing tissue damage. If however there are excessive free radicals present (due to a diet rich in fats or sugars, cigarette smoke, alcohol, chemical pollution, etc.) and inadequate antioxidant nutrients in the body (vitamins A, C, E, B, selenium, etc.) then the process can get out of hand and tissue damage may result. This process is now thought to be the starting point of many cancers (the free radicals can damage the genetic blueprint of the cell, the DNA, thus causing it to mutate), as well as the atheromatous changes in blood vessels which are the beginning of cardiovascular disease, and also of aspects of arthritis. Certainly in rheumatoid arthritis some of the inflammation involves free radical activity.

Thus the same nutrients which enhance immune function are the ones which damp down excess free radical oxidation.

There have been attempts to find a dietary pattern which would limit such activity in arthritic conditions in general, and in rheumatoid arthritis in particular. One such diet involves the use of particular essential fatty acids, derived mainly from fish, but also found in plants.

Bowel Health and Arthritis

As indicated in earlier chapters, the element of food sensitivity, or actual allergy, is often considered to be a part of the process of inflammation in arthritis. Such processes often involve what is called malabsorption, in which partially digested proteins are allowed to enter the bloodstream from the bowel, due to changes in the bowel's structure and function, which may go back to infancy. It is found that in weaning from the breast there is often an intolerance to some of the early foods introduced, especially cow's milk. For a variety of reasons humans cannot always tolerate the milk of other species, and cow's milk seems to be a particularly difficult food to cope with.

Other early problem foods include grains, which along with milk are fairly recent additions to the human diet. These were only introduced to the human diet in any quantity within the last 10,000 years, and man's digestive capacity having spent some millions of years without these substances, has shown a particular reluctance to accept them, especially in infancy. They play a major part in allergies in general, and in food intolerance and malabsorption in particular. Many rheumatoid arthritics benefit from eliminating grains and dairy produce from the diet.

There are other elements to consider in thinking about bowel health. We have living within us billions of micro-organisms which are vital to our health. Most of these inhabit the intestinal regions and there, in return for accommodation and food which we provide, they perform useful services such as synthesizing certain vitamins and generally assisting in digestive function. This intestinal flora, as it is called, changes with the type of diet we follow. One which is rich in fats and refined starches (sugars, white flour products, etc.) can be shown to compromise the flora severely, in its normal functions, and health suffers as a consequence. Again, free radical damage may be involved and there is a likelihood of such a diet producing a degree of constipation. In such a condition undesirable breakdown products remain too long in the bowel and can irritate the lining and cause local changes. For these and other reasons, malabsorption problems (intake into the bloodstream from the bowel of undigested or partially digested protein and other particles) often result, and these can relate to inflammatory processes such as rheumatoid arthritis. The intestinal flora may also be severely compromised by the use of antibiotics, which destroy large amounts of friendly bacteria along with whatever else it is being aimed at. A substance called serotonin is produced by the body when foods to which we are sensitive enter the system. This is involved in the inflammation within the joints of rheumatoid arthritis.

The type of diet recommended in this book will enhance bowel function and intestinal flora health automatically. This could be further enhanced by the use of acidophilus concentrates. These are some of the friendly bacteria, and repopulation of deficient colonies is possible by the judicious use of high quality acidophilus products. By paying attention to the adequate presence in the body of antioxidants (vitamins A, C, E, selenium, etc.) and ensuring desirable essential fatty acids such as EPA, as well as taking care of bowel health, there is a reasonable chance that we can control rheumatoid arthritis. All the methods outlined in the sections dealing with exercise, self-massage, trigger point treatment and especially hydrotherapy are also helpful for rheumatoid arthritis. Stress-reduction methods and the use of positive thinking also add to the body's chance of coping with the problem, and none should be neglected.

Some other specific factors of value in all arthritic conditions, including osteo- and rheumatoid arthritis, are outlined below. Firstly we should consider that remarkable nutrient antioxidant, selenium.

Selenium and Arthritis

The mineral element selenium is a truly remarkable substance, being of value in the protection of the heart, as an anti-cancer agent and of value in arthritis, as well as having numerous other benefits to offer. Norwegian studies have shown that selenium levels in the body were low in patients suffering rheumatoid arthritis, and that this was reducing the efficiency of a protective enzyme in the body called glutathione peroxidase. Such patients benefit from selenium being added to their nutrient intake. In osteoarthritis it has also been shown that supplementation with selenium reduces pain to injured and damaged joints, especially when combined with other antioxidant supplements, such as vitamins A, C and E (there are a number of combinations of A, C, E and selenium available). The same benefits noted in humans are found in animals suffering from arthritic joints, when selenium and vitamin E (they act synergistically) are given. Selenium's major role is as part of this powerful team of antioxidants, and as an enhancer of vitamin E. Consult a nutritionist or your health care provider for a recommendation of daily doses of selenium and vitamin E.

Vitamins and Arthritis

We have briefly discussed vitamins in previous chapters; the notes in this chapter are meant to expand on those specifically involved in inflammatory conditions such as rheumatoid arthritis, although most are of value in osteoarthritis as well. Both vitamin B_6 (pyridoxine) and vitamin B_5 (pantothenic acid) have been shown to produce beneficial effects on different types of rheumatic complaint.

B_6 is found to have the following effects; it decreases finger pain, as well as stiffness and numbness in the hand, shoulder, hip and knee areas, and helps to prevent night-time cramps.

Vitamin B_5 has been used successfully in both osteo- and rheumatoid arthritis, in the form of calcium pantothenate. One of its prime roles is in promoting the body's own production of cortisone from the adrenal glands (see below).

Vitamin C and Arthritis

This versatile nutrient is a major part of the substance collagen (rheumatoid arthritis is sometimes called collagen disease). Collagen is the substance which comprises cartilage, the major shock-absorbing tissue in joints, which is destroyed in arthritis. Vitamin C together with minerals such as calcium and magnesium and the vitamins A and B, as well as amino acids such as proline, will help to rebuild damaged collagen. (See also the notes on glucosamine in Chapter 4.)

Natural Cortisone

These nutrients (mainly vitamins C and B_5) are important for the health of the adrenal glands, which produce the body's own cortisone. Adrenal function is depressed in arthritis, and is also impaired by stress of all sorts. Support with B_5 and vitamin C is therefore helpful in reducing the burden on the adrenal glands and helping them to function normally. The natural production of cortisone carries no side-effects, but its introduction as a drug does.

Bromelaine and Cysteine

Whilst not strictly a nutrient, bromelaine is a remarkable extract of a common food, pineapple, although the form which is produced commercially of this remarkable enzyme is derived from the stem of the plant. It was first introduced in the late 1950s and it is reported to have a wide range of activities including aiding digestion, being a relaxer of smooth muscle and an inhibitor of blood aggregation (i.e., it keeps blood the right consistency) aiding in cancer prevention and being an enhancer of wound healing. Above all, from the arthritic's viewpoint, it has major anti-inflammatory benefits with virtually no side-effects.

Bromelaine is useful in all cases of tissue inflammation, and this of course includes most arthritic conditions. Since it is virtually non-toxic, bromelaine may be used almost ad lib, unless there is any sensitivity or allergy to pineapples. It comes in doses of 200 mg; 1 or 2 such tablets may be taken 3 times daily to aid inflammatory processes. These should be taken away from meal times, or the enzyme will become involved in digesting the meal (it is a protein-digesting enzyme). Its pain-relieving benefits are the result of its action to reduce local swelling and inflammation, and not of any direct painkilling ability.

Its activity in the body is enhanced, and indeed activated, by the simultaneous taking of manganese. Taken daily (1–3 g) for a month – together with vitamin B_5 and vitamin C in the ratio of one part cysteine to three parts C – will provide maximum benefit. People with diabetes should not take cysteine, but in all other cases of chronic ill-health, and rheumatoid arthritis in particular, it is recommended. After one month reduce the daily dosage by one third, and after a further month reduce this by another third, always keeping the ratio with vitamin C of 1:3.

Histidine

In many cases of rheumatoid arthritis it is found that there is heavy metal toxicity, such as aluminium, cadmium, lead, etc. This in itself leads to free radical activity, as well as other harmful effects. An amino acid fraction of protein called histidine has been used in the US in doses of 6 grams daily to good effect in cases of rheumatoid arthritis. Interestingly the Russians use this for their cosmonauts as a part of anti-radiation protection.

Amino acids are available from health stores.

Glucosamine sulphate, discussed in Chapter 4 should also be considered in rheumatoid conditions.

6

Herbal and Other Natural Remedies

A number of substances, some herbal and some derived from marine organisms, have been found to alleviate the symptoms of the arthritic patient. Such products include extracts of New Zealand green-lipped mussels and deep water sharks. Some of these have remarkable effects on the symptoms of pain and inflammation. In discussing aids and comforts to the symptoms of arthritis it is essential to bear in mind that nothing that these substances do is capable of making the condition worse, as is the case with some pharmaceutical drugs. There is of course no harm in disguising symptoms, such as pain (unless the usefulness of pain to prevent the undesirable overuse of an inflamed or damaged joint is thus obliterated so that the joint is then overused and damage increased).

Many herbal substances can help in a variety of ways. One of the most potent of these is the African herb Herpagophytum procumbens, better known as 'Devil's claw'. This can be obtained as a tea or as a tablet, and in many cases provides a means of eliminating acidic wastes, thus improving the condition of an arthritic joint. Use of this, or any other herbal method, should be accompanied by the use of the detoxification diet explained earlier. The herbs discussed below are also helpful.

Alfalfa contains vitamins, minerals, trace elements, eight digestive enzymes and eight essential amino acids. It therefore rebalances the glandular system as well as the blood. It is well known in the US as an arthritis aid. Burdock root is another useful herb. It is one of the best blood purifiers, and helps to break down cholesterol and calcium deposits, and neutralize poisons. It is especially useful for reducing swelling in joints. Also useful is celery seed, which is a strong diuretic and has a high mineral content. Its penetrating oils make it a powerful remedy for rheumatism.

Uncaria Tomentosa, commonly known in English as Cat's claw and in Spanish as Una de Gato, is a vine found wrapped around the trees in the rainforest of Peru. Historically, Una de Gato was used by natives as a tribal medicine for arthritis, gastritis, cancer and other diseases. Recent research suggests that the constituents of Cat's claw may contain properties that aid the digestive and immune systems.

Apart from immune enhancement and antioxidant properties, Cat's Claw often benefits arthritis. And European studies have determined that Uncaria Tomentosa has very low toxicity even if taken in large amounts. This may be of interest for those individuals suffering from painful joints who are unable to take medication due to side-effects.

Contraindications: Una de Gato is contraindicated for transplant carriers because of possible graft rejection. During pregnancy or if nursing, Una de Gato should not be used.

Suggested dosages: For prevention as an adaptogen and antioxidant, 1 to 3 grams daily in divided doses if using capsules, or 1 to 2 cups if using tea. For therapeutic use, 3 to 6 grams or 4 cups of tea daily.

Comfrey root contains the powerful healer allantoin, which helps to repair blood vessels and eases internal pains. It cleanses both the intestines and the blood.

Another useful plant is kelp, which promotes glandular health. It particularly helps the thyroid and adrenal glands. It concentrates the supply of vitamins, minerals and trace elements from the sea, and gives the body the chance to produce most of the enzymes necessary for the removal of rheumatic and arthritic deposits.

Finally, sarsaparilla is useful as a blood cleanser, and is specific for rheumatism. It also helps with glandular balance through its supply of natural hormones.

All herbs mentioned are obtainable from health food stores or herbal shops. They can be used either individually or can be made up into mixtures by a qualified herbalist in order to promote the functions indicated in their descriptions.

In a number of trials, both green-lipped mussel extract and squalene (an extract from deep water sharks) have been shown to be capable of relieving arthritic conditions, sometimes to a remarkable degree. These should be avoided, however, by those who are sensitive to fish.

These self-help methods in treating arthritis offer relief, and short-term gains, but do bear in mind that long-term benefit relies on the removal of the causes, whether they be physical, nutritional or emotional.

7
Stress and Emotional Factors

It is now well established that many forms of ill-health are directly related to our habitual thought patterns. Our consistent thinking patterns create our experience of life, and this can directly affect the ways in which we become ill. We have already discussed some of the ways in which habitual posture, as well as inadequate exercise, may contribute towards joint problems. We are also aware of the possibility of doing something positive through our eating habits, to assist the body to cope better with the stress of life. In terms of our emotional and thinking patterns we need, if possible, to identify those areas which may be contributing to the overall dysfunction of the body. If we only knew what was underlying our problems, we could take action.

The work of Louise Hay in the US has identified particular thought patterns that often precede, or accompany, arthritic conditions. Those that cause most general disturbance include a tendency to be over-critical of others, of oneself and of life in general. Emotional states which most frequently promote arthritis include bitterness, resentment, criticism and a general feeling of being unloved. Rheumatism is often accompanied by feelings of resentment, chronic bitterness, a desire for revenge and a lack of love and affection. All of these emotions can be released from consciousness and, with practice, replaced by compassion, forgiveness and love.

We have to go beyond the merely physical to the mental causes of our states of health. Using the relaxation and guided imagery methods described earlier and inserting positive thought patterns such as, 'I have compassion for others, and for myself: I accept joyful feelings,' we can begin to replace negative feelings. Whatever has gone before must be put aside, and we must become aware of our potential for health and happiness and realize just how much this depends upon our attitudes. The concepts that are most helpful in replacing the worn, old, habitual, negative thoughts and images include the uplifting ones of love, peace and joy. Love of others and of self has enormous healing power. It dissolves anger, releases resentment, dissipates fear and opens the way to health and harmony. Louise Hay writes the following as an example of the sort of positive affirmation of these ideas:

Deep at the centre of my being there is an infinite well of love. I now allow this to flow to the surface. It fills my heart, my body, my mind, my consciousness, my very being, and radiates out from me in all directions and returns to me multiplied. The more love I use and give, the more I have to give – the supply is endless. The use of love makes *me feel good*; it is an expression of my inner joy. I love myself, therefore I take loving care of my body. I lovingly feed it, and my body lovingly responds to me with vibrant health and energy. I love myself, therefore I provide for myself a comfortable home, one that fills all my needs and is a pleasure to be in. I fill the rooms with the vibration of love so that all who enter, myself included, will feel this love and be nourished by it. I love myself, therefore I work at a job that I truly enjoy doing, one that uses my creative talents and abilities, working with and for people, that I love and that love me, and earning a good income. I love myself, therefore I behave and think in a loving way to all people, for I know that that which I give out returns to me multiplied. I only attract loving people in my world for they are a mirror of what I am. I love myself, therefore I forgive and totally release the past and all past experiences and I am free. I love myself, therefore I love totally in the now, experiencing each moment as good and knowing that my future is bright and joyous and secure, for I am a beloved child of the universe, and the universe lovingly takes care of me now and forever more. And so it is.

This is something which might be read and repeated many times to help to cancel past thought patterns, and to replace these with a guiding principle and ideal.

In general terms the following aspects of daily living could also be examined to see if lifestyle and behaviour are contributing negatively to current health problems.

1. Avoid working more than 10 hours daily and ensure that you have at least one and a half days a week free of routine work. If possible an annual holiday 'away from it all' is advisable.
2. During each day have at least two relaxation or meditation periods. Time should be set aside morning and evening, or just prior to a meal.
3. Perform active physical exercise for at least 10 minutes daily, or for 20-minute periods 4 times each week.
4. Balance the diet and eliminate stress-inducing foods and drinks.
5. Try to move, talk and behave in a relaxed manner.
6. Seek advice about sexual or emotional problems that are nagging away at the back of your mind, or which are causing conscious anxiety.

7. If there are stress-inducing factors at work or home, which can be altered, then take concrete steps to eliminate these.
8. Cultivate a creative rather than a competitive hobby, e.g. painting, DIY, gardening.
9. Try to live in the present, avoiding undue reflection on past events or anticipating possible future ones.
10. Concentrate on whatever the current task is, always finishing one thing before starting another.
11. Avoid making deadlines or 'impossible' promises that could lead to stress. Take on only what you can happily cope with.
12. Learn to express feelings openly in a non-belligerent way and, in turn, learn to listen carefully to other people.
13. Accept personal responsibility for your life and health. Do not look outside yourself for causes or cures, apart from the objective guidance and practical advice available from a professional health practitioner.
14. Greet, smile at and respond towards people in the way that you would like to be treated.
15. Introduce negative ionization into the home or work place and ensure adequate exposure to full-spectrum light.

Some of the ideas that have been looked at can be used positively to assist in dealing with underlying emotional or attitudinal habits, which have become fixed. These in turn may affect our physical well-being. Thus, changes in thought may lead to changes in the body and so diminish the prevalence of arthritis in our society. Self-help begins with awareness, and with acceptance of oneself. From that point progress is possible, and indeed probable.

Index